CHUBSTER

CHUBSTER

*A Hipster's Guide to Losing Weight
While Staying Cool*

Martin Cizmar

MARINER BOOKS
Houghton Mifflin Harcourt
Boston New York 2012

For information about permission to reproduce selections from this book, write to Permissions, Houghton Mifflin Harcourt Publishing Company, 215 Park Avenue South, New York, New York 10003.

www.hmhbooks.com

Library of Congress Cataloging-in-Publication Data
Cizmar, Martin.
Chubster : a hipster's guide to losing weight while staying cool / Martin Cizmar.
p. cm.
ISBN 978-0-547-55934-6 (pbk.)
1. Weight loss—Popular works. 2. Low-calorie diet—Popular works.
3. Exercise—Popular works. I. Title.
RM222.2.C489 2012
613.2'5—dc23   2011028554

Book design by Lisa Diercks
Typeset in Belizio and AG Book Rounded

Printed in the United States of America
DOC 10 9 8 7 6 5 4 3 2 1

For Kirsten

CONTENTS

CHUBSTER

PROLOGUE

THE WORD *CHUBSTER* — WHILE UNIVERSALLY ACCEPTED AS SO delightful that it has to have *some* meaning — is fairly amorphous. Actually, UrbanDictionary.com, the definitive source of information on made-up words, offers quite a few definitions, two variants of which are interesting to us:

1. Chubster

(Noun)

An overweight person who considers himself to be a hipster. Someone who is proud to be a fatty mcfatfat ... They wear Old Navy jeans because they can't fit into anything from Urban Outfitters or from trendy thrift shops. They try to squeeze themselves into small hoodies and H&M T-shirts because slim-fitting clothes look "dope" on them. They avoid being an outcast loser because they are seen as cool and desirable due to a magnetic personality and funny jokes that compensate for their perceived lack of physical attractiveness.

Celebrity examples of Chubsters: Jonah Hill, Zach Galifi-anakis, Seth Rogen

Fawn: Ugh! Look at that chick with the muffin top and those Charlotte Russe flats.

Ruby: . . . and you know she got that Run-DMC T-shirt from Torrid.

Fawn: Oh em eff jeez, she's such a chubster.

2. Chubster

(Noun)

Someone who used to be chubby when they were a kid, but became very in-shape, muscular, and attractive. It's almost like being a chubster is a compliment, because most of them are very nice, they know what it's like to be the fat kid who's everyone's friend, no more (girls didn't think of him that way), so most chubsters don't judge. He's the guy who everyone likes, but how could you not like a chubster? Funny, nice, and able to relate to almost everyone? They're one of a kind.

Bob: Dude, this new kid came to our class, he showed us his yearbook and he was like majorly chubby two years ago.

Sally: But not anymore. That new kid's cute, that chubster.

For much of my life, I've been a Chubster[1]. Certainly, I was not seriously ashamed of my weight, and I was kinda-sorta proud of my indulgence. At the same time, I was always trying to fit in with my usually-skinny hipster friends—not always easy for a big guy. Now I'm working on becoming a

Chubster²: the cool, formerly fat guy. Actually, in calling this book *Chubster,* I'm hoping to carve that definition into a metaphorical stone tablet. Not that I'm always a nice guy—as you'll undoubtedly see throughout the book, I've never been the sweet and beloved tuba-playing fat kid—but I'm trying. I'm *trying,* folks. In the meantime, I'm doing what I've always done, which is keep it real. That means giving you some cold, hard, and unpleasant facts. I'm going to do that in the nicest and most efficient way possible because I've been in your shoes. I'm now an average weight, but luckily I still have some of that renowned empathy that makes fat people beloved the world over.

The fact of the matter is, there's nothing wrong with being fat. Or, at least there's nothing wrong with you *because* you're fat. That's the truth, and anyone who tells you differently is an asshole. Sure, I lost 100 pounds in eight months for the express purpose of *not* being fat (I'm 5'11" and weighed 290 when I started). Still, I don't see anything wrong with being overweight, per se. It's not a character flaw. Being fat is pretty fun, actually. I had a great run. I ate creamy, fried, and sickeningly sweet foods so delicious, most of my thin friends could never imagine consuming them. I imbibed mass quantities of the world's most delicious beers without a second thought—never did anything less caloric than Blue Moon touch my lips. I sat around playing video games, watching football, and listening to records on lazy Sundays. Despite my girth, I had no trouble getting a little action from attractive girls (my girlfriend is 5'10", a size 6, and gorgeous), which is the major impediment faced by the overweight among us.

Honestly, it was great. Sure, I was a little ashamed at the pool, but not enough to change anything. And there was that one time I could not fit inside a roller coaster. Only the Insane Clown Posse seemed to sell concert T-shirts that fit me. And I hurriedly untagged almost every photo of me posted on Facebook. But that was my life and I was enjoying it.

But "happily fat" is not a sustainable lifestyle. Facing my twenty-ninth birthday, I had to accept that. It was a cherry Slurpee and my girlfriend, Kirsten, which made me see this. It's sort of a weird story, actually. We were headed home from a Dave Matthews Band concert—part of my job is to go to such concerts and explain to the primitive hordes why they suck—when I stopped for a refreshing, sugary beverage to quench my thirst and propel me through the late-night writing process required to meet my 9 A.M. deadline. I got the largest size and sucked down the whole thing without a second thought. Kirsten, a nurse who works with liver patients, some of the least-well humans on earth, was horrified. We'd talked about my weight before, but never very seriously.

I could tell immediately this conversation was going to be different.

"DO YOU KNOW HOW MANY CALORIES YOU JUST DRANK?" she asked. I guessed around 300—it's mostly ice, right? When we looked it up (a ritual I would become all too familiar with in the coming months), it was more like 600. Some 600 calories for a bedtime snack! It was a lot, but still, I didn't see the big deal. Maybe a Slurpee was a bad choice, I said, but I need to drink something to write. How am I supposed to write with a dry mouth and tired eyes? Diet Coke, she suggested. Ick, I said. *No,* she said, *this is serious.*

The health thing, obviously, was a big concern. But the probable consequences—to be outlined shortly—also felt far into the future. There was a more pressing issue: In a few months, I would be meeting her health-nut parents for the first time in New Zealand. Kirsten's dad is a college professor who studies pharmaceuticals, and her mom knows everyone in her town's co-op grocery store by name and does nearly as much yoga as Gandhi—in other words, they've been granola since before it was cool. I knew Kirsten was right. There was little chance I could plan to be indefinitely overweight and keep that little pink heart on my Facebook relationship status intact. For me, it wasn't so much an ultimatum as a realization.

And thus began the transformation. A hundred pounds. A snug 44 to a loose 34. A loose 3XL to a snug M. Some people might prefer I say I dropped the weight with the help of Whole Foods, reusable BPA-free water bottles, and an elliptical, but the truth is, I didn't. I changed my habits so little that I might think it was pathetic—a sign that I'm pitifully stuck in my ways—if it weren't for how inspiring the story seems to be to other people.

If you're already supermotivated to lose weight, perhaps you should skip ahead to the first chapter now. This plan will work, I promise you that. If you're planning to lose weight and were drawn to a book like this in the store, that's really all you need to know to get started. But if you're a little unsure about things, read on. This is my attempt at giving you the Nudge. The best way I can think to do that is by telling you about my Nudge, which came from YouTube.

The day after the Slurpee Incident, Kirsten sat me down to watch a YouTube video wherein a medical professor gives a lecture about the various maladies caused by obesity. I don't want to ruin the end of the movie, which you can find at ChubsterTheBook.com, but (SPOILER ALERT) the fat guy dies. Just kidding. He mostly just suffers. Among the terrible health consequences outlined were:

- high blood pressure
- diabetes
- cancer
- high cholesterol
- arthritis
- sleep apnea
- premature death

Though I'm sure some people will disagree, for me, death was the least scary item on that list. The scariest? Diabetes. My dad has diabetes. It was diet-controlled for years, but he's now on insulin, which means needles are involved. Eek. My paternal grandmother had diabetes—she had a leg amputated before her death, which came when I was only a toddler. Double eek.

Sleep apnea was a little scary too, since one of my relatives sometimes sleeps hooked up to some kind of iron lung prescribed after a sleep study confirmed he suffered from the condition.

And, come to think of it, heart disease was a little worrying, since half my antecedents keeled over from massive coronary failure, including my rail-thin and very frugal grandfather, who had a heart attack after a handyman presented him with an unexpectedly large bill for a new water heater.

Actually, cancer too, since my mom has metastasized breast cancer, as did her older sister, who recently passed away. Scary.

Arthritis brought on by the strain your joints endure as

they propel your extra heft around? Not so scary. I mean, if you're seriously obese, you probably won't live long enough to make your odds dramatically worse than what heredity hands you. And with my genes, why worry, right? Given all the other grim health consequences I was facing, knee problems later in life seemed pretty trivial.

"I love you, baby, and I want you to be around," Kirsten said.

"I don't want to give you insulin injections when you inevitably become a bloated diabetic" is what I heard her say.

I took a deep breath and committed myself to losing weight, just as you must. Then I sat down to figure out the other really challenging part—the plan by which I could accomplish it. You don't have to do that, obviously, since I did it for you and wrote a whole book about it. (In addition to this book's advice, you may also want to seek out that of a doctor.)

When and how did I come up with the plan? Well, I came up with it immediately after agreeing to lose the weight. And I did it because I could not find an acceptable alternative.

The conversation went something like this:

"So, what are you going to do to lose the weight?" Kirsten asked.

"What do you mean?"

"I think you need to join some sort of program so you'll be accountable and so you have some structure."

"Ugh. No way. That just sounds awful. I'll do it. I know I can hold myself accountable—and that you'll hold me accountable, anyway—and I'm not joining some stupid group. That sounds expensive and lame. Paying money to hang out with a club of fat strangers in sweatpants debating whether Chunky Monkey or Cherry Garcia is more tempting? No thanks!"

"Well, I think you should join a group for support. And some sort of gym."

"I'm definitely not going to the gym. I don't have the money and I would definitely hate it—it's just a bunch of spray-tanned douchebags. Do I look like I want to hang out on the Jersey Shore?"

"Well, you need to do something. You can't just do this on your own; it won't work," she said.

"Look, I'm open to doing something, just so long as it's, you know, cool," I said. "I don't want to feel pathetic—people who pay to join stupid groups to solve their problems are pathetic. I want to do this my own way. Some way that's pretty chill, ya know?"

"There's no cool way to lose weight."

"Ummm. There's gotta be."

Here's my guarantee: This plan will be effective and you will not feel like a loser doing it. It won't always be easy, but it's not that hard, either—and it's a lot easier than submitting to the horrors of Organized Dieting. The Chubster plan is not only the Least Awful Diet Plan of All Time, it's the only plan for those who consider themselves cool.

You will not have to go to the gym, but you will get some exercise. As with any remotely plausible diet, you can "eat any food you want," though I'll take you through all the operative corollaries and caveats.

I'd hesitate to say, "If I'd have known it would be this easy, I would have done it a long time ago," since, as I said, being fat was fun. But if you've picked up this book, you're probably already interested in making the big change. So suck it up and hop on the bandwagon.

I'm going to make a token case for why you should lose the

weight in the first chapter, then I'm dropping it. You need to find that motivation on your own. I will say, however, that losing weight is a lot easier than the scum suckers behind the $60 billion Organized Dieting industry would have you believe. And, as you'll see, weight loss can be done gracefully and on the cheap.

I'm not really here to encourage you to do it; a girlfriend or a YouTube video—or, in my case, both—are better suited to that task. But if you're going to do it, you might as well do it this way. The cool way. The Chubster way.

We[2] are owning "Chubster," starting now.

ROCKET SCIENCE: SOMETHING CALORIE COUNTING IS NOT

God does arithmetic. —CARL FRIEDRICH GAUSS

HERE IS A QUICK TRICK FOR IDENTIFYING AN ORGANIZED Dieting scam intended to separate you from your money without providing any actual assistance: Look for the phrase "without counting calories" somewhere in the promotional material.

Look, I know calorie counting has gotten a bad rap. *It's such a hassle! I hate numbers! I hate having to think about everything I eat!* Blah, blah, blah.

Is counting calories fun in any traditional sense? Well, no—not for you and me, anyway. Is brushing your teeth fun? No, but is there a better way of preventing tooth and gum disease? You brush your teeth because it's the best way to take care of your mouth, and you're going to count your calories because it's the best way of shrinking your belly. Period. So it doesn't sound as fun to you as eating a plate of Atkins-friendly bacon? Boo-fucking-hoo.

Maybe there's a legitimate reason people loathe counting calories. Perhaps it has something to do with outdated notions about how hard it is to come by the information needed to calculate the calories in what you just ate—which we'll address fully later. Maybe. Call me a kook, but I fear it has a lot to do with an attitude fostered by Organized Dieting. You know: Big Slim. Fonda's Folks. The South Beach Mafia. *The Man.*

Honestly, I'm not above claiming that this crusade against calorie counting is a conspiracy. Calorie counting is so simple and so effective that it's a real problem for the $60 billion weight-loss industry. If you can count calories, you can lose weight while eating "whatever you want" because you can expend more energy than you take in. It's that simple, which is why there's a lot of money to be made muddying up the concept, often trying to restrict calorie flow while disguising it as something else purportedly much more complicated.

I mean, look at Weight Watchers. First, let me just say that I know Weight Watchers has been effective for a lot of people. Believe me when I say some of my best friends are on Weight Watchers. I'm not against Weight Watchers; it's just not for me. Or people like me. Hey, if you're looking for a lot of structure and some uncomfortable emotional encounters with obese strangers in stretch-top pants, they can probably help you. But you should probably know that the traditional cornerstone of the Weight Watchers program—the proprietary formula they call Points—is not all that different from good old-fashioned calorie counting.

The Points system is presently in disarray. At the end of 2010, the company tossed out its long-standing formula for one that's much more complex and geared toward promoting fresh fruits and veggies over processed foods, prompting a backlash from loyal customers. Under "PointsPlus," four elements—protein, carbohydrates, fat, and fiber—are all used to assign a point value to a particular item. Oh, unless the item has alcohol or sugar alcohol in it, in which case it's on a separate system altogether. It's enough to make you weep for the good old days when we calculated points using just calories, fat, and fiber!

The new formula is a trend-conscious gambit, but it's still all smoke and mirrors. According to the *New York Times,* the company's data suggest that "while members ate different foods, their caloric intake was roughly the same." Lo and behold, the results seemed to be about the same too, with the company making the flimsy boast that customers would lose "at least as much if not more"—"if not" being the operative weasel phrase. Either way, the company is facing a revolt over the switcheroo, and it's too early to see if it'll stick. My guess is no.

First, because, as it's worth pointing out, when people get adjusted to it they can easily overindulge. Under the new system, fruits like apples and bananas are zero points. A banana has about 100 calories, however, so if you add three or four a day, that "at least as much" could quickly become "almost as much" or "still a little." I honestly don't think PointsPlus is long for this world; maybe it'll even have gone the way of New Coke by the time you're reading this.

So let's look at the formula the fifty-year-old company used before that. Under the literally patented classic Weight Watchers system you've heard about for years and years, a point is calculated using the number of calories in the food, adjusted down based on how much fiber there is or upward based on how much fat there is. The formula actually looks like this:

$$p = \left[\frac{c}{50}\right] + \left[\frac{f}{12}\right] - \left[\frac{\min\{r,4\}}{5}\right]$$

In other words, points equals the number of calories divided by 50, plus grams of fat divided by 12, minus grams of fiber (up to and including 4 grams but not more) divided by 5. I should point out that you should not actually use this formula for any practical purpose; the company insists that would violate intellectual property law. The formula's existence is a matter of public record, but its use is forbidden without permission. Not that you'd have to do the math yourself, of course, since Weight Watchers has a million ways to give customers this information without requiring them to do any math. This is part of the program's allure and has the capitalism-friendly side effect of making customers feel dependent on the program. It's much better to be independent and use good old-fashioned science yourself.

Practically speaking, the traditional Weight Watchers formula means that because of the calorie-counting base, counterbalanced by fat and fiber, a Big Mac (590 calories) and a McDonald's Low-fat Asian Chicken Salad (714 calories) are both 14 points, which encourages you to eat a little healthier as you budget your calories under threat of extreme hunger. Slick, right? The problem is that, whether calories take the form of tofu or pork chops, you're not going to lose weight if your body doesn't actually burn them. Even if all you take in is salad, you need to use more than you take in to create the deficit that makes you lose weight. In fact, I'm pretty sure I could play with the numbers enough to figure out a way to *gain* weight on the old Weight Watchers while staying within my points. I'm absolutely positive I could do so on the new system, which would allow me to eat six bananas a day with impunity—a scenario that's not quite as outlandish as it might seem. Either way, I'm definitely not hugging some lady in sweatpants to prove my point.

Maybe this will seem a little shady to you, but when I've had to retroengineer a calorie count based on Weight Watchers' points on a restaurant menu (I'm not sure whether Weight Watchers pays places like Applebee's for the privilege of quantifying the healthiness of a handful of menu items or vice versa), I just multiply the number of points by 50. That technique gets close to the number of calories in the salad, though it definitely overestimates on the burger, which doesn't bother me too much.

Considering it's patented and all (again: that formula is for looking at, not for calculating with! Please respect Weight Watchers' intellectual property rights!), you'd figure the formula would be a panacea for weight loss. Sadly, a study (funded by Weight Watchers, no less) in the *Journal of the American Medical Association* found that the average person following the Weight Watchers Points program lost an average of 6 pounds in two years. Those who made it to about four-fifths of the weekly meetings lost an average of 11 pounds in two years. Pathetic.

Or, as Dr. Stanley Heshka, the scientist in charge of the 2003 study, said the customers' weight loss "is not very much in comparison to what people hope they will lose, or what people need to lose in order to reach the desired, svelte self."

Why would anyone put themselves through this pricey and ineffective program? Why not cut out the middleman?

In my research, I tried to pinpoint the origin of the phrase "calorie counting" and track its evolution so I could figure out when it, like the word "liberal," became saddled with such a harsh connotation that it's nearly impossible to use positively. Sadly, my *Oxford English Dictionary* and Google were not much help. Google's news archives were a little edifying, though. Let's look at this blurb from Kansas's *Kiowa News,* a press release from the American Medical Association reprinted on January 18, 1968:

> Calorie counting is a favorite pastime of those of us who want to lose weight. The term "calory" is used in a unit in expressing the energy-producing value of food. When we say that a tablespoon of honey contains about 100 calories, it means that the honey, when utilized by the tissues of the body, will release that amount of energy to be expended by bodily activity. The usual weight-reduction goal of one or two pounds lost per week is achieved by an average daily intake of 500 to 1,000 calories less than needed to maintain the weight at which reducing was begun.

That's actually pretty much 100 percent right, as I'll explain further. Even forty years later, with all of our so-called advances and quick fixes, the advice in a small-town Kansas newspaper is still the most accurate.

It may feel as though I'm beating you over the head with this, but I want to be clear: You will count your calories and you will like it, or you will put this damned book down right now and go back to stuffing cheeseburgers down your gullet. Counting calories does not have to become "a favorite pastime," as the AMA suggests, but it's absolutely the fastest and most effective way to lose weight.

The Bagel Paradox

If you're going to make any headway with the weight-loss thing, you're going to need to understand something I call the Bagel Paradox. Honestly, I hesitate to name this phenomenon after the worldwide mascot of Jewish food, given the long history of tragedy suffered by the Twelve Tribes, but it's really the perfect example. So, here goes: Bagels are evil. Please don't hear this as anti-Semitic. Many of my best friends are Jews. Some of my best friends are Jewish deli heirs. But that doesn't make the bagel any less evil.

The problem with the bagel has nothing to do with a lack of deliciousness, certainly. As savory baked breakfast goods go, I'd probably put them on top, above the muffin, English muffin, or muffin top. No, the issue with bagels is that people think they're healthy—which they aren't, at least not for dieters. Grainy and unglazed though they may be, bagels are always calorie intense and thus a treat for the dedicated Chubster in the making. If you're going to lose weight, you're going to have to give up—or at least curtail your consumption of—so-called healthy foods like the bagel, which contain way too many calories to let you lose weight.

Just do the math.

Take an Einstein Brothers' sun-dried tomato bagel, which, just like the plain bagel, has about 320 calories. A Krispy Kreme Original Glazed has only about 200 calories. Well, you're thinking, the bagel has tons of good stuff in it, like fiber. How can I go wrong? Sure, the bagel has 4 grams of fiber, but even the doughnut has 1 gram. Actually, back when Krispy Kreme was still offering their whole-wheat Original Glazed, it was arguably nearly as healthful, with 2 grams of fiber in 180 calories. Yes, a doughnut with roughly the same calorie-to-fiber ratio as a bagel. It existed, once.

And those figures are without any sort of topping. Dough-nuts don't need toppings, at least not where I come from. But bagels do. Toss on four tablespoons of plain cream cheese (which you very likely will between the two sides of the bagel), and you're adding 200 calories (or another doughnut). So, yes, for the same number of calories you can have three Krispy Kreme originals or one bagel with cream cheese.

Now let's toss in a regular chai with skim milk—sounds healthy, right?—which is 190 calories. That's equivalent to another doughnut and black coffee. Four doughnuts with coffee or one bagel with cream cheese and a skinny chai: your choice. Obviously I'm not saying that four doughnuts is a good breakfast for someone trying to lose weight; I'm just saying that a bagel and cream cheese isn't any better.

The thing is, most people don't look at food this way. Not when they're eating, not when they're judging the habits of others. Take it from a man who has eaten both a bagel and three doughnuts in front of coworkers: no one blinks an eye at the bagel, while three doughnuts could very well trigger a response from HR about abuse of the company health plan. Fat, sugar, and fiber matter, sure, but from the strictly weight-oriented perspective of a calorie-counter, these two choices aren't so different, at least not in the way people think.

The first step toward an easily manageable weight-loss process is learning about how many calories are actually in your food. To do that, you desperately need to eliminate much of what you think you know about "healthy" foods and use this book as a jumping-off point for discovering low-cal foods you'll enjoy that can fill you up and meet your nutri-tional needs. Later chapters will deal with this subject in depth; now it's enough to know that you'll need to get beyond the Bagel Paradox. Before we get to "how," we need to get to "when." It's time to set some goals.

Your Number(s)

Ideally, you'll see a doctor about losing weight before embarking on any program, including this one. I did. I got a check-up about 35 pounds into my program (with a full panel of blood tests my girlfriend ordered, with the consent of a doctor, to make sure I was "not already diabetic") just so I could be positive I wasn't messing anything up. I'd strongly recommend you do so, too. A doctor could probably fill in the numbers you'll read about below in a microsecond. However, to honor the DIY spirit of punk rock fanzines like *Maximum RocknRoll,* Ian MacKaye, and that run-down rental house near the campus that was always hosting shitty basement shows, here are all the relevant facts and figures.

First, you need a final goal. I picked something nice and round—100 pounds—then set to work. It doesn't have to be such a big number. Doctors typically determine whether you're at a healthy weight based on something called the body mass index (BMI), which puts an individual's height and weight on a sliding scale, then attempts to deduce how much body fat you have based on those figures. Technically, even at 190 I was slightly "overweight," based on BMI. As it happens, I have an especially long torso and stubby legs, a trait that artificially inflates many people's BMI, in some cases costing them unduly large health insurance premiums.

It's actually a major problem. The many evils of BMI are described in a number of books and articles, and I suggest you check out *The Obesity Myth,* in which University of Colorado law professor Paul Campos rails against BMI as a tool of corrupt insurance companies and government agencies. He points out that, according to the government's BMI standards, Brad Pitt is overweight and George Clooney is obese, which should raise your eyebrows. Still, BMI is the easiest way to get a rough estimate of what you should weigh, so go to ChubsterTheBook.com for the BMI calculator. That and some common sense should help you figure out an appropriate target weight. From there, the rest of the process is pretty straightforward.

A pound of body fat is made up of about 3,500 calories. So to lose a pound of body fat, you'll need to create a calorie deficit equal to that amount by burning more calories than you consume over a matter of days or weeks. If you want to lose a pound a week, you'll need to create a 500-calorie deficit every day for seven days. If you want to lose 2 pounds a week, you'll need a calorie deficit of 1,000 calories a day. And so on. Generally, it's considered unhealthy to lose more than 2 pounds a week, though plenty of diets suggest it. If you're very, very obese, as I was, you could lose more than that just by eating the so-called typical 2,000-calorie diet, while someone who is, say, only 20 pounds overweight would have a totally different diet plan from the start.

The trick, then, is to calculate how many calories you typically use in a day to figure out how many fewer you need to eat to create the desired deficit, keeping in mind that 2,000 calories is the FDA's typical diet and that going too far below that could be dangerous or counterproductive. Talk to a doctor before doing anything, especially anything crazy.

So, how many calories do you burn in a day? That's best figured using the Harris-Benedict principle, which will give you your basal metabolic rate (BMR)—the amount of calories you burn by breathing and such. There are about a zillion websites and computer programs that'll do this for you, and ChubsterTheBook.com has the hook-up, of course, but just for your edification, BMR goes by this formula:

Women: 655 + (4.3 x pounds) + (4.7 x height in inches) - (4.7 x age in years)

Men: 66 + (6.3 x pounds) + (12.9 x height in inches) - (6.8 x age in years)

Activity is also a factor. If you're sedentary, multiply your BMR by 1.2 to determine how many calories you burn in a given day. If you're very, very active, multiply it by 1.6. If you're somewhere in the middle, pick the appropriate spot on the continuum between 1.2 and 1.6 and multiply it out.

Now you know how much you could eat in a day to maintain your weight where it is. Subtract 500 from that, and you'll know how much you need to cut to lose a pound a week. Subtract 1,000 to know what you'd have to eat to lose 2 pounds. And so on. Pretty simple, right? As I said, this is not rocket science. It's also not patented. This is just good old-fashioned, nonproprietary, totally foolproof science.

Here's how it worked out for me: When I started my diet, I was way, *way* overweight, so the pounds just kept peeling off. Essentially (since my numbers looked like this: 66 + 1,827 + 915 - 190.4 = 2,617.6 x 1.2 = 3,140), I could eat 3,000-plus calories a day and *maintain* my weight. Yes, that's right. I could eat Big Mac Value Meals (1,170 calories each with the sandwich, medium fry, and regular Coke) for both lunch and dinner and three Krispy Kreme original glazed doughnuts for breakfast *and lose about a pound a week.* I could have *lost 2 pounds a week* by switching those Cokes to Diet Cokes. Insane, right?

I chose to eat just a little over half that crazy number, 1,800 calories, which is not too far below the "normal" 2,000-calorie diet, putting me in position to lose about two and a half pounds a week before considering exercise. At the beginning, there were times when I actually lost 5 pounds in a single week, which makes sense given my numbers. That decreased over time, even as I increased the intensity of my exercise regimen.

I adjusted my weight goals depending on how quickly I was progressing, but I always aimed for around 2 pounds a week after the initial plummet. My goals tended to be focused on holidays and trips, working back from the final goal: 100 pounds before the New Zealand trip in January. For example, before my family vacation, a cruise to Alaska in July, I wanted to be at 255. Before a backpacking trip in early September to Havasupai, a remote part of the Grand Canyon, I planned to be at 225. I wanted to be at 210 by Halloween and 200 by Thanksgiving. At the risk of sounding too girly, I must confess that, for further motivation and to gauge my progress, I also made a habit of picking up slightly small "goal shirts" at thrift stores, planning to wear each when I could fit into it—more on that in later chapters. As I said, perhaps that's something even *Glee*'s Kurt Hummel wouldn't do if he mysteriously found himself fat, but it worked for me. Sometimes I blew by the goals weeks early, sometimes I struggled until the last day, but each time I managed to clear the bar.

What about your goals? That part is personal. Meeting my girlfriend's parents in some sort of respectable shape was my big goal, while my ten-year high school reunion, at Thanksgiving, was not a factor at all. As I met my buddy for drinks at a pub that night, it did occur to me that I was thinner than I had been in high school, but I didn't care enough to actually show off. Maybe you'd feel the opposite. Whatever you do, though, be sure to start with a target weight-loss figure, then divide it by a reasonable weekly goal to see how long it should take you. Then look for some milestones along the path. You'll be standing at the end of the trail in no time, and it'll actually be a pretty pleasant trip (thanks to the rest of this book).

You're welcome.

TOOLS

Man is a tool-using animal. . . . Nowhere do you find him without tools; without tools he is nothing, with tools he is all!
—THOMAS CARLYLE

WHY IS DIETING SO HARD AND COMPLICATED? OR, RATHER, why do people think it's so hard and complicated? I think it's in large part because dieting is a pretty new concept—in the grand scheme of things, at least.

Think about it. Evolution has finely tuned the human body for the lives of tribesmen engaged in hunting, gathering, and subsistence agriculture. Our ancestors lived that way for millions of years, and, of course, a fair number of people around the globe *still* live that way. Sorry to go evolutionary biologist on you here, but your body's natural inclination is to get and store whatever fat you can because you never know when a hard, cold, and hungry winter is coming. Gaining weight is a natural tendency. When you diet, you're actually subverting your body's hard-wiring.

This is why widespread obesity is a thoroughly modern phenomenon. For most of humanity's existence, people had to work too hard to get too fat, and the people who managed to pork up were society's elite, more or less viewed with awe by the skinny and unwashed masses.

Dr. Benjamin Caballero, a Johns Hopkins University professor, considered this topic in a very special obesity-themed issue of the Oxford journal *Epidemiologic Reviews.* He blames The Man. You may or may not find that comforting.

> For centuries, the human race struggled to overcome food scarcity, disease, and a hostile environment. With the onset of the industrial revolution, the great powers understood that increasing the average body size of the population was an important social and political factor. The military and economic might of countries was critically dependent on the body size and strength of their young generations, from which soldiers and workers were drawn. . . . Historical records from developed countries indicate that height and weight increased progressively, particularly during the 19th century. During the 20th century, as populations from better-off countries began to approach their genetic potential for longitudinal growth, they began to gain proportionally more weight than height. . . . By the year 2000, the human race reached a sort of historical landmark, when for the first time in human evolution the number of adults with excess weight surpassed the number of those who were underweight.

So not only did the Millennium coincide with the Official Rise of Fatness, we're fat because Ford Motor Company and the U.S. Army needed stocky cogs in their evil industrial war machine!

Bum bum bummmmmm!

Chances are, you're a little too caught up in the task at hand to appreciate this, but pause for a moment and consider the wonderfulness of our current predicament: Every social class in America can get fat. It's unparalleled in history. Sure, probably a few Americans starve to death every year, but that's more than likely not because of scarcity. More likely, it's because they do something like set off into the Alaskan bush with only a rifle, a book about native plants, and a journal, planning to live in an abandoned school bus until discovering that the animals are wily and the poisonous and safe plants look an awful lot alike. That's pretty much what it takes to starve to death on American soil these days. If you manage to do it, there's a fifty-fifty chance Jon Krakauer will write a book about you.

You get the idea: Our plenitude is a major accomplishment! Caballero goes on to call our ability to produce an abundance of dietary energy "one of the major achievements in human evolution." That's right, fatness is a byproduct of *"one of the major achievements in human evolution,"* according to a man who has a Ph.D. in neuroendocrine regulation from MIT.

You don't even know what neuroendocrine regulation is, do you? Neither do I. In fact, I looked it up and I still can't explain it beyond stating that it has something to do with how your brain interacts with your glands.

The point is this. Caballero is really smart, so when he puts your obesity in a larger context, accept that what he's saying has some real weight (pun not intended) and that you are not "fat" but "evidence of a landmark accomplishment by our species."

Fatness is a byproduct of the leisurely life your hard-working ancestors and the greatest minds of the Western world have been working to create for millennia. They wanted you to have a life of plenty, a life without backbreaking work. Your great-great-great-grandfather would weep with joy at the sight of you half-conscious on a couch, having just shoveled a pile of fried noodles straight out of the takeout carton into your mouth after a busy day organizing the office's fantasy football league. *Surely my descendant has become a king!*

Yes, our overweight society is, by the standard of the ancients, a utopia. You've relished it, taking full advantage of your ability to eat like a devout hedonist at an all-inclusive resort while neglecting to tax your muscles with arduous labor. Of the billions of people who've ever lived, you have it easier than almost anyone. History congratulates you.

But as the Notorious B.I.G. once remarked, things done changed. Alas, our well-fed workforce fell victim to the Law of Unintended Consequences. Having binged on cheap and readily available comfort food until they ballooned to epic portions, Americans started falling victim to the unpleasant consequences of obesity.

Things got even worse as the percentage of people making their living by manual labor decreased. The burger/fry/milkshake thing was fine when a large percentage of Americans worked in factories, but not so much after the changing economy picked them off the assembly line and plunked them down in cubicles. Alas, burgers, fries, and milk shakes are no less delicious—and most of the restaurants serving them have thus far had little market incentive to evolve into healthier establishments—so society continues to slip farther down the spiral.

Sure, the undernourishment of olden times had its fair share of unpleasant side effects, but there are also a wide range of undesirable consequences of a plump populace.

Back to Caballero:

> Although obesity did not attract the attention of the mass media until recent decades, its prevalence in industrialized countries began to increase progressively early in the last century. By the 1930s, life insurance companies were already using body weight data to determine premiums, having identified an association between excess weight and premature death.

D'oh. They've known about this since the 1930s? That's not even a decade after White Castle invented the concept of the fast-food hamburger chain! This feels eerily reminiscent of that whole smoking-cancer thing.

The First Dieter

Actually, the first well-known diet predates that time. No sooner had the industrial revolution given rise to fatness than someone sought to fix it.

Enter William Banting, an Englishman who wrote the first widely read "diet book," a pamphlet called *Letter on Corpulence Addressed to the Public,* way back in 1862. Banting's open letter documents his struggles with "corpulence" (the old-fashioned term for fatness) and recommends a simple, straightforward eating plan.

Great, right? Forward-thinking scholars and other public scolds must have loved this guy! He must have been a cherished celebrity, the Jared Fogle of his day!

Eh, not so much.

Though his name was synonymous with dieting (literally, people actually called the weight-loss process "banting" for years), Banting became the target of "ridicule, contempt, and abuse" from "men of eminence" (read: nineteenth-century doctors and scientists). They called his eating plan "humbug," though they themselves had no idea how obesity might be cured by other means.

In 1865, a leading London newspaper even ran a hit piece quoting prominent members of the British Science Association who wanted to debunk Banting's diet, which called for limiting heavy, fatty foods and carbs. The general public was much more forgiving, though, taking quite a shine to his informal essay, which, to postmodern eyes, somehow manages to be both stuffy and touching:

> Of all the parasites that affect humanity I do not know of, nor can I imagine, any more distressing than that of Obesity, and, having emerged from a very long probation in this affliction, I am desirous of circulating my humble knowledge and experience for the benefit of other sufferers, with an earnest hope that it may lead to the same comfort and happiness I now feel under the extraordinary change—which might almost be termed miraculous had it not been accomplished by the most simple common-sense means.

Heartwarming, right? Like a lot of dieters, Banting started with stupid ploys recommended by know-it-all friends. He tried rowing for a few hours in the morning, but the vigorous activity just made him hungrier, and he actually gained weight. He turned to medicine, looking for a no-effort, quick fix. The crap he took, liquor potassæ, thankfully did nothing, which is still about the best you can hope for with some crazy pill-based diet advertised on late-night AM radio today. Turkish baths were in vogue, so he tried to sweat off his fat. He was, of course, unsuccessful. Finally, he found a doctor who told him to limit his consumption of butter, bread, sugar, beer, milk, and potatoes. That worked splendidly.

Remember, odd as it sounds, this was before doctors made the connection between the massive consumption of rich foodstuffs and weight gain, so this was hardly obvious advice.

Unfortunately, Banting's plan was also the first gimmick diet—there was, for example, a total prohibition of potatoes, milk, and beer. It wasn't exactly well balanced, but it succeeded in cutting calories (along with a few things it didn't need to cut), so it worked.

Happily, dieting quickly became much more sophisticated. Within a few decades, a chemist named Wilbur Olin Atwater used a "calorimeter" to burn various foodstuffs, then carefully measured the leftover ash to determine how much energy was contained in each item. The concept of food calories was born, and the connection between high-calorie foods and weight gain was soon established. *If you take in more energy than you use, your body stores the extra energy as fat? Oh, that makes sense!*

Atwater's protégé at Wesleyan University, Francis Gano Benedict, continued his research. In 1918, he coauthored *A Biometric Study of Human Basal Metabolism,* which contained a formula known as the Harris-Benedict equation. (Maybe the name of that formula looks familiar from the first chapter of this book?)

At that point, the fundamental rubric for successful weight loss was established.

Everything else is epilogue. The facts were scientifically established; applying them is the art.

That very year, Dr. Lulu Hunt Peters, a California physician, took calorie counting mainstream with a book called *Diet and Health*. Her plan, which was geared exclusively to married, middle-aged women, was pretty basic: Just eat a dozen 100-calorie portions every day. Her book was a huge hit and sold a staggering 2 million copies, thanks to its friendly and familiar tone and simple instructions.

"Hereafter you are going to eat calories of food. Instead of saying one slice of bread, or a piece of pie, you will say 100 calories of bread, 350 calories of pie," Peters scolded.

Lulu, it's fair to say, had a little of the Chubster spirit in her. ("If there is anything comparable to the joy of taking in your clothes I have not experienced it," she once wrote.) The one-size-fits-all 1,200-calorie plan worked for people to varying degrees. Looking back, the most useful thing in Peters's book was probably a table of the number of calories in foodstuffs, information that was not widely available at the time.

We can only imagine the reaction of the primitive, naive creatures reading this astonishing information for the first time, their faces betraying puzzlement, excitement, and doubt.

Cal-o-rees? How positively titillating!

Still, it's all there. Should you desire, it would be perfectly feasible to procure one of the eminent Dr. Peters's tomes and follow its advice.

What's the point of all this historical context? Partly, to show that your obesity is not solely your personal failing but part of a global trend that predates your birth by a century. That's not an excuse; it's historical fact. Also, to illustrate that you have no excuse for not counting your calories.

Normal people have been successfully counting calories for ninety years, back when looking up nutrition information required a trip to the library and low-calorie microwave meals were the subject of science fiction. You've got it pretty damned easy, kiddo. If ever you should find yourself complaining about the task of looking up the calories in restaurant food online and logging it into the electronic device in the palm of your hand, I want you to picture your grandfather silently shaking his head in disgust, ashamed at how lazy and stupid his progeny has become.

▦ The Metric System

If you travel overseas during your diet, as I did, you may encounter the kilojoule. Think of it as a "metric system calorie." Now, you could go native, recalculate your daily food intake in kilojoules, and download a new app for your phone, but I find it easier to do the conversion. There are 4.1868 kilojoules in each calorie, so multiply the number you find on the back of that triangular Toblerone box by four and you've got a calorie figure to work with.

Here's the deal: Counting calories is an easy, two-step process. First, you need to figure out how many calories you're eating. Second, you need to make some record of it. That's not so hard, right?

Know what's even better? You can totally tailor your counting method to your lifestyle so you don't damage your image in any way. One of the great things about the Chubster plan is that it lets you choose between Hi-Fi and Lo-Fi options, from the iPhone to an old-fashioned Moleskine notebook.

Chances are, you cringed a little when reading either "iPhone" or "Moleskine." That's normal. Most of you will find one of those things indispensable (or at least desirable) and the other useless, annoying, and overpriced to the point of being gauche.

It's all good, guys. While there are a lot of people who use the word "hipster" merely as a derisive term for "annoying young person wearing current fashions I don't like," as you probably understand, it's a lot more complicated than that. Hipsters come in a wide variety of flavors, each with unique proclivities. Their tastes and interests tend to overlap in a number of places (Arcade Fire, American Apparel, PBR), but hipsterdom is in no way born of a hive mind.

Actually, to the untrained eye it might be possible to think a lot of hipsters belong to another subculture entirely. A lot of hipsters-gone-green sorta look like regular, run-of-the-mill hippies. Some *Arthur*-reading hipsters ironically enjoy Swedish death metal so much, you might suspect them of being actual metalheads.

You're not fooling anyone here, though. In order to build a calorie-counting plan, we need to determine which of five insufferable caricatures of hipsterdom most resembles you. Stereotype yourself, and we'll handle the rest.

You are: Music Snob Hipster

You are seen: At record stores, dive bars, and club shows staged by buzzing indie rock acts.

You wear: Ironic concert T-shirts for '80s hair metal bands or cheap brands of domestic beer. Not only are these still kinda cool, the original nonironic fans of those bands and beers also tend to be overweight, so it's easy to find something in your size.

You carry: A USB turntable and a cardboard box full of 78s.

You read: Pitchfork. Sometimes you slum it with Stereogum.

You work as: Probably a bartender who DJs when you can get gigs. Maybe a record store clerk or bank teller.

Your friends are: The people you see at shows. You may also have some other acquaintances you try unsuccessfully to get to go to shows.

You got fat because: You felt yourself putting on some weight after college, and your original plan was to follow the advice on that Brooklyn Vegan blog all your friends were talking about. There's actually nothing about food on there, though, and you instead got sidetracked. You spent the next three years downloading mp3s and stuffing your face with microwave burritos. Also, that trip to Portland, when you ate at every one of Beth Ditto's favorite spots, didn't help.

You will get nutrition information from: The best and most efficient way, which is to Google "calories in [insert food]" and go with the first or second result unless it seems really fishy. By varying your sources, you decrease the chance of getting the sort of consistently bad information that'll undermine you. You probably don't eat that many new or exciting foods anyway—you're too busy keeping abreast of the developments in other areas—so it won't be a constant struggle.

You will count calories using: Back issues of *NME*. Just kidding. You'll use a simple app for your out-of-date cell phone or, if you're really analog, a few slips of paper you keep in your purse or wallet along with one of those tiny pencils you use to keep score when playing miniature golf.

You are: Artsy Fashionista Hipster

You are seen: At gallery openings, museum fundraisers, hot DJ nights, and the occasional electronica show.

You wear: It changes from week to week. Are you still doing that arty apron thing, or is that as passé as hand-knit scarves? What about leggings—are those still in? Aviator sunglasses are finally out, right?

You carry: Glossy magazines featuring photos of pretty people looking sad in expensive clothing. A handbag that matches your shoes. The cell phone that is always attached to your ear in public.

You read: Fashion blogs, celebrity tweets, and Gawker.

You work as: A consultant for something or other. Pitch-person for new brand of exotic liquor. You sell stuff on Etsy.

Your friends are: Younger and thinner than you.

You got fat because: This is a tough question because few mortals have actually seen you eat a full meal. Maybe it was too much free food and liquor at industry parties. Maybe you just ate at too many hip new restaurants. Keep in mind that there are more than 125 calories per ounce in foie gras, so even sharing an appetizer hits hard.

You will get nutrition information from: You probably know in advance where you'll be eating since it is the coolest newest place and everyone is talking about it. You'll have to look at the menu in advance and Google the dish you intend to order.

You will count calories using: You could probably just use your phone, but if that seems a little too unstylish, try a vintage electronic organizer. An old 32kb Casio or Radioshack model is pretty small, even by contemporary standards, and will set you back only about $20. They look pretty cool—in an '80s sort of way—and you'll grab everybody's attention when you whip it out at a party. A vintage Trapper Keeper from the "Designer Series" (think: holographic flamingos, M. C. Escher knockoffs) is also a totally great look, but it's pretty big to carry around every day, so it's a serious commitment.

You are: All-Natural Hippie Hipster

You are seen: At the farmer's market or co-op. At the Phish show now that Animal Collective and Vampire Weekend said it's OK to like them.

You wear: Tom's Shoes (with every pair you purchase, they give a pair to a child in need!) and a flowing skirt or some sort of linen/hemp/organic cotton pants.

You carry: A reusable grocery bag from an appropriate retailer.

You read: Musty books about politics, religion, and philosophy. *Mother Jones.*

You work as: A perpetual student. A clerk at a kiosk in the neighborhood farmer's market.

Your friends are: That crazy old dude you see on the bus every day who you're trying desperately to turn into a wise old man you can talk to about your problems. People who aren't annoyed by your holier-than-thou lifestyle. The lady who makes that yummy organic avocado and olive oil dip you always buy and eat without sharing.

You got fat because: Brown rice is not less caloric than white rice. Also, you tried to go vegetarian but ended up eating way too much cheese and putting on a few pounds. Then you briefly went vegan but ate a half jar of peanut butter daily (there are 1,500 calories in a cup of that stuff, if you can believe it!) to get enough protein. You're back to free-range chicken and grass-fed beef now, but the damage is done.

You will get nutrition information from: Carefully reading the back of every item you buy at the co-op. Remember to look at the "servings per container," since a lot of "healthy" foods exploit the portions per pack loophole to give people a false sense of security. For produce and bulk foods without labels, just ask StarBlossom, Coyote, or whoever happens to be manning the front counter—just don't get suckered into buying a bunch of high-calorie brown rice.

You will count calories using: A notebook made from that horrible gray recycled paper. Be mindful of what you're buying, as some notebooks marketed as using "recycled paper" contain only about 30 percent postconsumer materials. Look for something like AMPAD Envirotec's wirebound notebooks, which are made from 100 percent postconsumer waste. Then, start each day by writing down how many calories you get for the day, subtracting as you go.

You are: Nerdy Bookworm Hipster

You are seen: At the library, bookstore, coffee shop, and other places where cool, well-read people congregate to talk about smarty-type stuff.

You wear: Frumpy sweaters to cover your bulges. Luxurious leather shoes you hope will distract people from the rest of your body. Eyeglasses.

You carry: A big leather bag with reading materials in it and a cup of cappuccino.

You read: Everything. All the time.

You work as: Grad assistant. Copy editor. Barista who aspires to be a writer.

Your friends are: Classmates and former classmates.

You got fat because: You hate "sports," "the gym," or "going outside." Also, you just had to try making some of Emily Dickinson's legendary dessert recipes so you could report back to the professor who wondered aloud whether the Belle of Amherst's gingerbread is really as incredible as is claimed in literary circles. It was purely an academic exercise, we understand.

You will get nutrition information from: A big, thick reference book. Having one on hand would be a hassle for most people, but when you're already lugging around a copy of Pynchon's *Gravity's Rainbow* and the latest editions of both *McSweeney's* and the *New Yorker,* it doesn't seem so bad. The latest offering from the CalorieKing series would probably be the most useful, but it's also a little too commercial. Look for Barbara Kraus's *Dictionary of Calories and Carbohydrates,* first published in 1974 and now in its fifteenth edition, instead. Or try to score a vintage edition of the *Pocket Guide for Calorie Counters,* published in the 1940s. True, those out-of-print reference books won't have a lot of useful information about today's foods, but they sure are cool and interesting.

You will count calories using: A Moleskine notebook and a fountain pen. You will make copious notes on each item, perhaps even using adjectives like "splendid" and "marvelous."

You are: Interwebber Tech-Geek Hipster

You are seen: Usually as an avatar or artfully cropped profile picture that minimizes your fatness. Occasionally at the Apple store.

You wear: A custom-made T-shirt with some sort of techie reference on it. A sport coat. Designer jeans in the largest size you can find.

You carry: A shoulder bag with an iPad in it.

You read: The first 200 words of random blog posts your tweeps point you to—you lose interest after that.

You work as: Social media consultant. Your company's IT guy.

Your friends are: The 4,000 people who follow you on Twitter. IRL? N/A.

You got fat because: You try to do a Foursquare check-in from any restaurant your tweeps are talking about with some sort of wiseass comment about how it's overrated. Also, your ass doesn't leave your desk chair for more than an hour each day, which makes it really hard to burn off even the sushi you had at happy hour.

You will get nutrition information from: Either Live strong.com, Calorie-Counter.net, or CalorieKing.com. When you Google most restaurant foods, these are usually the first sites you find (and, let's face it, everything you eat comes from a restaurant). You're sure to develop a strong preference for one of them in short order. After that, you'll fiercely battle the people who prefer the opposite site and snottily correct any mistakes you discover in the comment section in pure troll fashion.

You will count calories using: An app on your smart-phone. Obvi. If you do that, be sure to get the simplest one you can find, not one that's always prompting you to reward yourself for exercise with an increased calorie allotment. Personally, I like to have separate apps for looking up nutrition info and counting. This is why I prefer a big ol' database like the CalorieCheck app and a separate, simple counting

app like Food Diary from Felt Tip, which was better before they updated it with a bunch of unnecessary features
but still gives you a nice countdown. Livestrong and Calorie Count (caloriecount.about.com) both have nice apps, and
their databases are pretty good too—pick which one you like
and defend it to the death.

So you probably don't fit neatly into any of these little boxes.
Hopefully you don't. Chances are, however, you saw something of yourself in one of the caricatures. Are you always
playing with your phone, annoying your friends and loved
ones by updating your Facebook status at totally inappropri-
ate times? That habit is going to play a part in your plan. Are
you more comfortable with paper and a pen? Then that's how
you'll do this. You need to look at the suggestions above—all
the gadgets and techniques available to you—and decide on
an appropriate course of action.

It's really not that hard to count calories—just figure
out the calories in whatever you're eating and record them
somehow—but it does take dedication. You need to come up
with a plan and stick to it.

Chubster isn't about one single, rigid method; it's about
finding the right plan for your lifestyle. You're going to complete this mission in your own style; this book is just arming
you to do it. Right now, we're turning you into a self-sufficient
dieting machine capable of functioning in any environment.
Using what you're learning here, you'll be able to diet under
any circumstances, up to and including a meal at Earth's
single least hospitable place for a cool person on a diet.

That is, of course, Fat Boy's Pork Palace in Brandywine,
West Virginia.

(FYI: A cup of grits without butter is only 150 calories.)

Your Mother's Meat Loaf

You know why no strictly structured diet program can ever work? Because of your mom and her wonderful meat loaf.

Now, obviously her meat loaf (or whatever equivalent special recipe your mom happens to make) is not especially healthy. Still, not only do you love that meat loaf, you love your mom, and you're not going to make her sad by turning down a reasonably sized serving of it. Does your diet allow for this situation? If not, it's destined to fail.

This is one big reason that calorie counting works and everything else doesn't. So long as you can get Mom to tell you roughly what's in that pan so you can estimate the calorie count, you're golden. You may have to eat a salad for lunch to save up calories for it, but that's a small price to pay for both a mother's love and a working diet plan.

Calorie counting is flexible in this way—which is why it works and other diets don't.

The Seven Habits of Highly Effective Calorie Counting

As you can see, how you retrieve and record your calories is pretty much a free-for-all. The method doesn't matter much, and it's not using any skills you didn't develop in kindergarten. Honestly, there are probably a hundred ways that would work so long as you can stick with it.

The rules for making sure you're staying on track aren't so flexible, though. If you want to make steady progress throughout the weight-loss process, it's extremely important to stay disciplined enough to hold yourself to these seven simple rules.

1. Each Day Begins at Midnight. There are going to be times when you'll feel hungry in the evening and want to borrow against the next day's calories. That's not recommended—not until you're pretty far along, anyway—and the best way to keep yourself honest is to start your new counting day when the clock says you should. It's a great way to balance wants and needs. If you're still really hungry at midnight, there's nothing wrong with dipping into the new day's allotment, but you'll be happier come morning if you can fall asleep instead. You'll be surprised by how easy it is to avoid evening snacking when you postpone it until after your typical bedtime.

2. Measure Everything Possible. If you don't already have sets of measuring cups and spoons, you need to buy them now. Trust me: It's one thing to eyeball "a cup or so of cereal," it's another to actually measure it out. Chances are, if you try to guess the amount of foods you're eating, you'll be a little too generous with your portions. At first blush it might seem overly strict, but accuracy in counting is key to hitting your calorie goals. It won't always be possible—unless you want to carry a tablespoon in your pocket and measure salad dressing at an Italian restaurant—but by measuring whenever it's reasonably convenient, you'll develop an eye for amounts that will serve you well when it's not as practical to be exact. When you're in your own kitchen, there's no excuse, though.

3. Round Up and Down to 10. Remember the rule about "rounding half up" you learned in elementary school? You're going to do that again, rounding up and down so all your calorie figures end in zero. That is, if something has 94 calories in it, you can count it as 90. If it has 95 or 96, you count it as 100. Maybe you like the idea of being as precise as possible, but it's not worth trying to be any more specific than this. If you can guesstimate your food intake to within 10 calories at every meal, you're doing pretty well.

4. Use the Best Information Sources and Cross-Check Your Calorie Information When Possible. There are dozens of websites and smartphone apps promising accurate calorie information. Most of them are pretty good, though it's amazing how estimates vary from source to source.

Let's say you just had some vanilla fro-yo for dessert—it's a tasty, low(ish)-cal dessert and doesn't seem to vary widely by source. This should be easy to get consistent figures on, right? Not so much. Let's look at the first page of search results . . .

CalorieCount.com says there are 117 calories in a half cup—a very specific number considering they don't give a source. MyFitnessPal says there are 73 calories in a half cup. LiveStrong.com says there are 89 calories in a half cup of Yogurtland's French Vanilla. LA's Pinkberry publishes nutrition information saying there are 29 calories per ounce, or 100 calories per half-cup serving. The same amount of TCBY's vanilla has 120 calories according to the company's information. One blogger who took on the subject, Froyogirl .com, says Menchie's has 168 calories per half cup.

So if you just had a half cup of regular vanilla frozen yogurt from a mom-and-pop store, what would you do? That's a hard question when one estimate is more than twice another estimate. You have to get all the information you can and go with your gut (pun not intended). You can also help yourself avoid reenacting that *Seinfeld* episode about supposedly nonfat yogurt by not going overboard with something that seems to be too good to be true.

From my experience, Livestrong.com and CalorieKing .com (which are usually the first two results on things I Google) tend to be pretty accurate. Try to look at both if you have time, especially if one seems a little shaky. Also, always trust a restaurant's own estimate above anything else. If they're wrong, you can sue them.

By the same token, I don't like using phone apps that integrate calorie counting and calorie estimating, precisely because they handcuff you into one source's estimate, and every source has some flaws. Find an app that counts the way you like it and stick with that. If you've got access to the Internet, it's always better to do a search in your browser, though it's handy to have some sort of information resource downloaded in case web access is not available or running super slow.

5. When in Doubt, Compare to Something Known. Like any hipster, I greatly prefer local restaurants to chains, but the big companies' ubiquity does serve calorie counters. It's not always easy to get nutrition data for popular menu items at national chains, but it's almost always possible with just a little sleuthing. Since most restaurant food comes from similar—or the very same—food distributors, you're usually pretty safe going with the information you find online for chains. While the divy little bar and grill down the street doesn't publish nutrition info for its chicken sandwich, it shouldn't be hard to compare it to something equivalent. Does the sammy they're serving look more like a Burger-King TenderGrill (aka BK Broiler) or an Applebee's Grilled Chicken Sandwich? How about that burrito at the little taco stand by your office? Is it more the foil-wrapped monsters at Chipotle or the smaller kind you see at Del Taco?

6. Overestimate If You Can't Know for Sure. There will be times you're just not sure what's in something you're eating. Maybe it's made with a secret recipe. Maybe a friend cooked it and it'd be awkward to ask. Maybe there's no real equivalent sold by a restaurant that posts its nutrition info. When that happens, try to overestimate. Since studies show that most people dramatically underestimate how many calories they're eating, chances are you won't really be cheating yourself out of anything. Also, if you're eating something that can't be easily estimated, chances are it's not very diet-friendly anyway. It's important to do what you can to keep yourself honest.

7. Build a Database. Does tracking down calorie information seem like a fair amount of work? It can be, especially at first. But how often do you revisit the same dishes, in the kitchen or at restaurants? Probably pretty often, which makes things much easier after a few weeks. Depending on the method for recording you've chosen, you should have some way of easily retrieving the deets on foods you've noshed on previously. If you're going with paper, either put a star next to things you're likely to eat again or start a separate list in the back of your notebook. If you're digital, keep a file, or a note, with the stats for favorite dishes handy. Sure, if you follow rule 4 you're going to spend some time cross-checking information, but you'll soon make that time up using your database, which is stocked with the best numbers you can come up with.

So that's how to count your calories. Strictly speaking,

that's all you need. As we'll see shortly, one guy used this information to lose weight eating mostly junk food, taking the "so long as you're counting, you can eat whatever you want" principle to an absurd extreme. But, of course, there's always an easy way and a hard way—and, as I promised at the beginning, Chubster is about teaching you the easiest, least painful way to accomplish your goal. We'll learn that nowish.

EATING PART I: A MACRO-LEVEL PHILOSOPHY OF FOOD

Gluttony is not a secret vice. —ORSON WELLES

BY THE YEAR 2020, THREE OUT OF FOUR AMERICANS WILL BE overweight or obese.

Well, at least according to a recent study by an international group called the Organization for Economic Cooperation and Development. It claims that 75 percent of the American populace will be busting the scale by the start of the next decade. Sounds pretty dire, right? Maybe a little comforting, too? After all, when fat people are the majority, they won't have to deal with any nettlesome social stigmas.

I don't buy that study for a second. First, it was conducted by economists, a field that has proven itself consistently terrible at predicting future trends even on its own turf. Remember when they saw a recession coming? Yeah, me neither. You know what they call a really, really smart economist? An investor.

Economists have been getting things horribly wrong since at least 1798, when Thomas Malthus predicted that the world would soon run out of food because humans reproduce more quickly than farming techniques could improve enough to feed them.

"The power of population is indefinitely greater than the power in the earth to produce subsistence for man," he wrote in an essay that, believe it or not, still informs articles written by "neo-Malthusian" economists today.

Contrast that with the catastrophe that Franco Sassi, a senior health economist at the OECD and the man behind the "Obesity and the Economics of Prevention" study, predicts.

"Food is much cheaper than in the past, in particular food that is not particularly healthy, and people are changing their lifestyles, they have less time to prepare meals and are eating out more in restaurants," he said when the study was released.

So, while disastrous food shortages are still a serious area of study for some economists, other economists are saying we're in danger because we produce *too much* cheap food? No wonder it's been branded "the dismal science."

Call me crazy, but I truly don't believe America's obesity epidemic is going to get worse by 2020. In fact, I think we're going to see a dramatic shrinkage in the American waistline—with the Chubster plan getting only a small part of the credit.

Things look dim now, I admit it. Already, two thirds of

American adults are overweight or obese. Fast-food restaurants are marketing both foot-long hamburgers and breadless sandwiches made entirely of meat and cheese. Cheesecake Factory sells something called Fried Macaroni and Cheese that, not surprisingly, has 2,000 calories—a day's worth. At least people know what they're getting into there. Starbucks sells beverages that provide a third of the average person's daily calorie allotment without anyone batting an eye. And we're scarily sedentary. Americans sit for an average of 56 hours a week, according to a poll conducted by the Institute for Medicine and Public Health. We move around so little these days that a few years back some physiologists even tried to invent a disease called Sedentary Death Syndrome to describe it, though the label didn't catch on.

All that aside, human beings have proven to be remarkably adaptable to changing circumstances. This fatness thing isn't working, and we, as a society, have too much intellectual and economic capital to let it continue to drag us down. Sometime in the next decade or so, we will see the obesity epidemic reined in significantly.

Let's go back to Dr. Caballero at Johns Hopkins:

> Historically, human obesity was commonly associated with gluttony and lack of self-control at the table. Thus, treatment and prevention approaches were largely focused on individual behavior. Over the past decades, however, as the obesity epidemic continued to advance in the United States, there has been increasing focus on the external determinants of energy balance. . . . [T]here is an increasing consensus among obesity experts that changing the "obesogenic" environment is a critical step toward reducing obesity.

The "obesogenic" environment Caballero discusses basically boils down to the suburbanized world where the majority of Americans live. They commute to work by automobile and eat heavily processed food from the chain restaurants clustered around their houses. They therefore gain weight. Ain't that America, home of the free . . . with little pink houses for you and me.

But we will evolve. Balance will be restored. I promise you this.

Foods will get lighter. I'm not sure how, but they will, perhaps aided by exotic new ingredients or by people's turning back to simple, organic foodstuffs. Maybe new laws banning trans fats, mandating menu labeling, or something similar will make a difference. Maybe schools will teach kids enough to change their habits. Something will push the pendulum back on what we eat. This is the nature of our civilization. For every cultural trend there's a countertrend—Bret Michaels gives way to Axl Rose who gives way to Kurt Cobain. Exercise will creep back into our routines. People will begin to understand what's actually in their food in terms of energy and how they have to limit their consumption or increase their activity.

By following the Chubster plan, you're just getting a jumpstart on the process a lot of your friends and neighbors are going to go through in the next decade. Mark my words: There's no way we get to the point where 75 percent of this country is overweight or obese. You're an early adopter, not an outlier.

This chapter is about the dieter's philosophy of food, and it will repeat a lot of things you've heard before. However, you've heard them before because they make sense, and you're still fat because you ignored them. Now is the time to change that. The Chubster plan isn't an exciting fad diet that promises to magically transform you with the power of some Amazonian extract. It is, however, the very best weight-loss information available presented in the least painful way possible.

Let's start with the calorie thing.

What is a calorie? Well, scientifically speaking, it's the amount of energy needed to raise the temperature of 1 kilogram of water by 1 degree Celsius. It's the standard unit of food energy in this country (we'll talk about the alternatives later), which means that it tells you how much energy your body can pull out of an ingested substance. If you were what biologists and anarchists called rewilded, you'd want to eat lots of calories to make sure your body had plenty of power. In your current state, you want to use more energy than you take in so you can burn up the excess. Obvi, right?

Proper nutrition is certainly much more complex than simply limiting calories, but calories are what will make you lose or gain weight. "But I want to have a healthy heart and strong bones, too!" you might be thinking. That's all well and good, but right now you've got to focus on losing weight if you want to succeed. Trying to change everything overnight is usually a recipe for failure. You need to get the extra weight off first, then you can balance your diet and get plenty of "good fats" and "whole grains" and all that jazz.

Fact is, if you lose weight you will get dramatically healthier, no matter what you eat to do it. That's not what a lot of diet gurus and nutritionists would have you believe, but it's true. It's science, even.

Maybe you remember reading about that college professor who lost 27 pounds eating Twinkies. His name was Mark Haub, and he's a professor of human nutrition at Kansas

State University. He proved this point beyond any reasonable doubt, as far as I'm concerned, documenting his experience on a Facebook page, Prof Haub's Diet Experiments, and becoming a media sensation in the process.

Here's the gist of his work: When his students doubted his contention that eating whole grains, lots of fiber, berries and bananas, and vegetables could still leave him overweight, Haub decided to limit his calories for ten weeks. The twist? Most of his calories came from the junkiest of junk foods: Twinkies, Nutty Bars, Star Crunches, Zebra Cakes, etc. Such treats have essentially no nutritional value, so to keep himself from getting sick, he also added a few daily servings of low-calorie, nutrient-rich foods like baby carrots, green beans, and celery as well as a multivitamin and a protein shake.

Not only did the Haubster lose 27 pounds in ten weeks, his body fat percentage dropped dramatically, his "bad" cholesterol dropped 20 percent, and his "good" cholesterol increased by 20 percent. He reduced his triglycerides by 39 percent. In case you don't know it, these are the traditional measures of heart-healthiness, and he improved them by eating snack cakes.

Not that anyone, including Haub, thinks you should eat Twinkies when you diet. Nor should you eat brown rice and olive oil with abandon.

"There seems to be a disconnect between eating healthy and being healthy," he said. "It may not be the same. I was eating healthier, but I wasn't healthy. I was eating too much."

The point is this: When it comes to losing weight, calories are what matters. If you want to lose weight, you need to limit them. Yes, *you can eat anything you want,* just like the spammers sending you junk mail claim! You just need to make sure the amount you eat conforms to your daily calorie allotment. So have that Twinkie—just be sure to log the 150 calories.

Is this too simple? Would you prefer some sort of "forbidden food" gimmick? That's what all the best-selling diets do, I guess, so we should probably get on board. Fine, you can lose weight if you follow the Chubster diet and don't eat gingerbread.

Yes, gingerbread is now strictly forbidden by the Chubster diet. So long as you don't eat gingerbread (and also stay within your calorie allotment), you will lose weight. But, if you cave and eat gingerbread (or go over your calories), you'll stay fat forever.

Satiety

While you can eat anything you want (except gingerbread) and lose weight, that's not the most effective plan. After all, even if they have the same number of calories, a snack cake is not nearly as filling as a bowl of popcorn.

The science of dieting is in the calories; the art of dieting is in what they come from.

The goal of wise dieters is to feel full while eating fewer calories. By understanding which foods will best meet your needs—low calorie but filling and satisfying—you'll make things a lot easier on yourself.

And so I introduce you to the Satiety Index.

In 1995 a group of Aussie scientists led by Dr. Susanna Holt published an article in the *European Journal of Clinical Nutrition* documenting which foods made people feel most full given the number of calories eaten.

It was a rather ingenious study. Holt and her colleagues got volunteers to compare 240-calorie portions of 38 common foods. The tasters didn't see what they were eating, and the foods were served in the same size chunks and at the same temperature. Two hours after they'd eaten, they were given access to a buffet, where the people conducting the study measured what they took and questioned how full they felt.

The Satiety Index is based on that study. A slice of white bread was set as the baseline and ranked at a Satiety level of 100. Foods more satisfying than white bread ranked above that; foods less satisfying fell below.

Look at how two breakfast foods compare: Oatmeal scored an impressive 209 (twice as filling as white bread) while a doughnut came in at a lowly 68. That's why oatmeal makes a much better breakfast for a dieter—it's a lot more filling for the number of calories you're spending on it. More nutritious, too.

The very highest ranking food? Boiled potatoes, which are three times more satisfying than white bread. Take that, Atkinsites! Not that all carbs fared so well, though. French fries are only a little more satisfying than white bread. The croissant came in dead last.

The study—a partial list is below and the full list of rankings is easily obtainable online—shows that the most filling foods generally have a lot of fiber, protein, and water. So if you want to feel full while dieting, that's what you should eat. Likewise, foods such as popcorn and lettuce are so bulky, they tend to fill people up. Beans and lentils are absorbed slowly, so you feel full longer after eating them. Fruits are generally good, but sugary bananas are fairly low while fibrous apples and oranges are very filling. Fatty foods are all pretty low in satiety.

Ever wonder why dieters gravitate toward salads, popcorn, and baked potatoes? Now you know. Not that you can trust conventional wisdom completely. Yogurt and granola are generally considered healthy foods, but they're high in calories and low in satiety. Not that they don't have a lot of fiber, protein, and water compared to their fat and carb content. Actually, yogurt won't make you feel any more full for the calories than jelly beans.

Combining filling, low-cal foodstuffs with the right mix of higher-cal, but intensely flavorful and possibly nutritious, ingredients is the true art of dieting. That's what I get into in the next chapter. In the meantime, there are a few other minor concerns to address.

🍽 Satiety

Here are the most satisfying foods, ranked on the Satiety Index:

- boiled potatoes
- oatmeal
- oranges
- apples
- brown pasta
- beef
- baked beans
- popcorn
- All-Bran cereal

Here are the least satisfying foods on the Satiety Index:

- croissant
- cake
- Mars candy bar
- peanuts
- yogurt
- potato chips
- ice cream

The Iffy Science of Metabolism

While I'm generally a firm believer in the simple, straightforward science of basic calorie counting, I know people want to work all the angles. When it comes to weight loss, that means tweaking up their metabolism as much as possible.

Now, as you've probably noticed, Chubster is all for using hard science established through decades of serious study conducted by the world's experts in their respective fields—with a few snarky jokes to keep things palatable. Truthfully, most of the facts and figures we're working with here were established in the nineteenth century. Poring through all this old-timey shit sometimes makes me feel as if I'm listening to the Decembrists on repeat. Hopefully it's working for you, though.

On the other hand, the study of metabolism—how fast your body breaks down and uses the fuel you give it—is far less advanced. A lot of the information you'll find out there about "boosting your metabolism" is hooey peddled by snake oil salesmen and witch doctors. It absolutely should not be taken seriously, especially if it involves a pill (read: *TrimSpa, baby!*). That said, there is some serious scholarship being done on how to manipulate your metabolic rate, but it's all quite complex and certainly far beyond the understanding of the idiots writing Examiner.com articles about the virtues of green tea extract.

It's *possible* that you can get a little extra edge by following the advice you'll hear spouted, but don't count on it. Our metabolic rate is generally something beyond our control. Sorry.

Here are actual facts about metabolism as supported by science. This is going to depress and disappoint some of you, I'm sure, but you're better off knowing the hard truth.

Maybe you'll see a twinkle of hope here. If something makes sense to you, give it a try. Just don't use any of this information as an excuse to stray beyond your calorie allotment. While metabolism (probably) isn't something you can control in a meaningful way, what you eat is.

You don't have abnormally slow metabolism. Yes, metabolism does vary somewhat among people. And there *is* a disorder called hypothyroidism, in which your thyroid doesn't pump out enough of the hormones that keep your metabolism moving. Some estimates say as many as 10 million Americans—roughly one person in thirty—suffer from that disorder, so it is a possibility you're one of them and just haven't been diagnosed. If you think you have an actual medical problem involving your thyroid (other symptoms include fatigue, depression, constipation, decreased libido), go to a doctor and get tested. Otherwise, shut up about it.

Quit trying to blame your fatness on your metabolism. Yes, you may know a few people who immediately burn off anything they eat. Sorry, you're not one of them. Studies suggest your metabolism is mostly the product of your genes and is set from birth. It's not going to be changed easily and safely. You just eat too much and exercise too little, and that needs to change.

No, seriously, your metabolism is fine. Get tested if you don't believe me! When people talk about metabolism, what they usually mean is their resting metabolic rate, or RMR. Your RMR, which accounts for the calories your body burns through vital biological processes like breathing and pumping blood, accounts for between 65 and 75 percent of your calorie expenditure.

Figuring out your RMR—essentially, the number of calories you burn just sitting around—used to be a long and complicated process overseen by a doctor, but there is now a gadget that can do it in about 15 minutes. You just sit still and breathe into a tube, and it tells you how many calories you're burning. There are several brands on the market (BodyGem is the most popular), and chances are a personal trainer, gym, or doctor near you has one. Call around. They'll probably charge you more than $75 for the test, at which point they'll confirm what I just told you: You don't have an abnormally slow metabolism, you just eat too much.

Adding muscle will help you burn a few more calories just sitting, but it's probably not worth the effort. Your RMR is in part a function of your muscle mass. Both fat and muscle burn calories while you sit around playing *Halo,* but muscle burns more. How much more is hotly debated. As with anything about metabolism, a wide range of educated people disagree strongly about how many calories static muscle burns per day. Toss in the uneducated people who have also chimed in, and finding the truth becomes like finding a needle in a haystack. Some people say more than 100 calories a day. Others say only about 6.

From the studies I've seen, it seems the "muscle burns lots of calories when still" phenomenon is mostly a myth. Sure, people burn more calories while putting on muscle mass, but that seems to be largely a result of the physical activity they did to get the muscle. Rather than seeing a steady correlation between lean muscle mass and RMR, we see an initial spike in RMR as the first muscle is built, which then plateaus. Claude Bouchard, a professor at Louisiana State University, told the author of *Ultimate Fitness: The Quest for Truth About Exercise and Health,* that muscle actually has a very low metabolic rate at rest. He says it's 6 calories per pound each day.

Let's be extra generous and assume that a pound of muscle burns an extra 15 calories a day. This means that if you bulk up with 10 extra pounds of muscle, you'll be burning a massive . . . 150 calories a day! That's about one and a half bananas. Not such a big deal, right? Also, putting on that much muscle is serious business. You could add up to a pound of muscle a week if you're hell-bent on beefing up with weight training and protein loading, but don't think that all that extra muscle is going to make a huge difference in your diet. If you really want to lift some weights and drink some whey, go for it, but you'd probably do better focusing on the diet instead, especially since body-building diets and weight-loss diets are often at odds.

Don't expect the kind of food you eat to influence your metabolism. Studies show that the nutritional composition of your food doesn't influence your metabolism. No, eating more or less fat, protein, or carbs won't make you burn calories noticeably faster. Sorry. Digesting protein and fiber may force your body to use a little more energy, but not enough to make a noticeable difference in your weight loss.

Starving yourself will sabotage your diet. Starving yourself is never a dieting solution, as I mentioned earlier. If you dramatically cut your calorie intake, your body may slow down your metabolism and go into miser mode, conserving whatever energy it can. Stick to the daily figures you came up with in the first chapter or risk going backward.

Spicy foods won't save you. Sorry, but smothering your food in Tabasco sauce and jalapeño slices isn't going to boost your metabolism significantly. You'll get a little jolt because spicy foods raise your body temperature, but it's nothing meaningful. Trust me, if superspicy foods helped you burn a bunch of calories, I should have never been overweight to begin with.

Green tea might give you a tiny bump. Green tea is still riding a wave of good publicity based on a 1999 study in the *American Journal of Clinical Nutrition,* which showed it helped metabolism. Despite the hype, the findings were rather timid: "Green tea has thermogenic properties and promotes fat oxidation beyond that explained by its caffeine content *per se.*" Yes, *per se.* The figures you'll see repeated over and over are that green tea boosted energy expenditure by 4.5 percent. What they don't tell you is that placebo caffeine boosted it by 3.2 percent. That's a 1.3 percent difference.

On the other hand, a 2008 study in the same journal found that drinking green tea before exercise helped a fair amount. Subjects were asked to work out for 30 minutes after drinking green tea, and their fat oxidation rate was 17 percent higher than that of people taking a placebo. It's worth noting that the control group was not given caffeine plus a placebo, which may have been a factor. Either way, it's safe to say that drinking unsweetened green tea or green tea extract might help boost your metabolism a tiny bit. Just don't expect any miracles.

Now, from reading between the lines up there, you may also realize that caffeine does tend to help increase metabolism. In fact, that's the main ingredient in a lot of over-the-counter diet pills. So, yeah, have some coffee, tea, or diet soda—just don't expect miracles and remember that caffeine is a mildly psychoactive stimulant with noticeable side effects. As a hopeless addict, I've paid the price on numerous occasions, so I'm reluctant to push it on anyone. But it helps a little, so long as you don't mind the attendant hassles of dancing with Mr. Groundstone.

Drinking cold beverages won't save you. Yes, your body does use a tiny bit more energy processing ice-cold water. No, it's not enough to make any real difference.

Water will help metabolism a little. Drinking enough water is key to dieting, and a possible boost to metabolism is just one benefit. Traditional wisdom holds that you should drink 64 ounces a day (old folks say that's eight 8-ounce glasses; you and I know that's two 32-ounce Sigg bottles), and that's a good habit to develop.

Although a small German study published in the *Journal of Clinical Endocrinology and Metabolism* shows that drinking more water seemed to boost metabolism, that's been challenged by a number of others since it was published. Even that study found that at best you might burn an extra 50 calories a day drinking a liter of ice-cold water, and that's taking into account the supposed benefits of both the coldness and the general healthiness of water.

Eating small and frequent meals probably won't help. You've probably heard that eating small, frequent meals will speed your metabolism up. The idea is that metabolism is stimulated because your body works harder burning the fuel as it comes in slowly. Seems to make sense, right? Maybe that'll help? Eh, probably not.

Though the oft-repeated advice is backed up by some studies, the supporting research was often the product of extremes—comparing someone stuffing their face full with an entire day's calories at once versus someone else eating twelve times a day. Experts seem to suggest six smallish meals (or three meals and three snacks), and while that very well might help you stay full throughout the day, don't expect much of a boost in resting metabolic rate (RMR).

Several studies comparing dieters consuming the same number of calories over three and six meals—including a 2009 study in the *British Journal of Nutrition*—found no difference in fat loss, appetite control, or the hormones that signal hunger and satiety. As the *New York Times* wrote in reporting on that study: "As long as total caloric and nutri-

---

♀🎥♂ Water

Drink 64 ounces of water a day? Yeah, that's just an old wives' tale. There's no scientific basis for the number, and no one knows where the estimate came from or how it became gospel.

Even the popular myth-busting website Snopes.com couldn't sort the story out fully before declaring that truism "False."

Should you be drinking more water? Maybe. However, according to a kidney specialist quoted in the *Los Angeles Times,* average adults in a temperate climate probably get enough fluid from the food they eat in a day to replace what they use or expel.

Still, you should probably try to drink more water while dieting. Here's why:

• Water fills your stomach, helping you eat fewer calories. A study conducted by a Virginia Tech nutritionist found that people ate between 75 and 90 fewer calories at a meal if they first drank 16 ounces of water.

ent intake stays the same, then metabolism, at the end of the day, should stay the same as well."

Typical exercise will give your resting metabolism only a small, short-term boost. Research shows that energy expenditure does not return to your normal baseline immediately after exercise. The bad news, however, is that if you're doing the typical 20 to 30 minutes of cardio, your body will be back to normal within an hour or so. Your kidneys and liver and lungs may use an extra 30 calories calming down, but that's all.

> • If you're drinking water, you're not drinking something with calories. Water, of course, has no calories. It's probably obvious that drinking regular soda or other sweetened drinks is one of the worst ways to spend your calories. A can of Coke has 155 calories in it, almost all of which are from sugar, and it won't fill you up much. True, diet soda offers an alternative, but if you have—or can develop—a taste for plain ol' water you're better off.
> • Your body works better with plenty of water. A great majority of the biological processes your body performs in a given day use water. It's necessary to remove waste products, carry nutrients, and regulate your body temperature. When you diet, you're trying to purposely put your body under some stress to make it burn off energy stores, so don't tax it further by not giving it enough of something it needs.
> • You should be exercising (more on that later), in which case you will need to replace the fluid lost when sweating.

Contrary to what you've been told dozens of times, your body doesn't continue burning more calories after you've stopped working out, according to a 2009 study in *Exercise and Sport Sciences Reviews*. This study involved both moderately active people and serious endurance athletes, and the results were the same: When you stop working out, you stop burning extra calories. Surprised? Don't feel bad, the guy who led the study said he was "flabbergasted" by the results.

"Bottom line is that we once thought that exercise would burn calories, especially fat calories, for a long period after a bout of exercise," the exercise physiologist Gerald Endress told MSNBC. "This does not seem to be the case."

EATING PART II: A MICRO-LEVEL LOOK AT STUFF YOU CAN (AND SHOULD) EAT

There are people who strictly deprive themselves of each and every eatable, drinkable, and smokable which has in any way acquired a shady reputation. They pay this price for health. And health is all they get for it. How strange it is. It is like paying out your whole fortune for a cow that has gone dry.
—MARK TWAIN

By now you know what you can eat on a diet: anything —except gingerbread—provided you don't go over your calorie allotment. Simple, right? But what should you eat? That's a more complicated question, indeed. We've taken a long time to get to this point, I know, and you've had to read a lot about science and other junk in the meantime. I'm truly sorry for that, but it was necessary to set the stage. Now, we'll sort out what you should be buying and consuming on a daily basis. That's the fun part, right?

The idea here is to find foods that delight, satisfy, and nourish you within your daily calorie allotment. That's tricky, because, as I said before, when you diet you're deliberately hacking around your body's hard-wiring to create an artificial scarcity, thereby forcing it to burn stored energy. Creating such a scarcity without feeling hungry is a challenge, since, ya know, that's how bodies tend to work. In fact, the whole idea of not being hungry on a diet is paradoxical—you are, by definition, restricting your intake below what you actually need to maintain your current state. Your body responds by telling your brain you're hungry. That's natural, though admittedly unpleasant.

An added challenge comes from social situations that involve food. It's a lot easier to make the right call when you're standing by yourself in front of the freezer than when you're looking at a big menu surrounded by friends and a busy waiter. When you're dining out, we want to put you in a position to make either smart or stupid—but not ignorant—decisions about what to eat. "Smart" is better than "stupid," of course, but both are way better than "ignorant."

The Chubster plan is all about losing weight gracefully, remember, and so our goal is to have you ordering just like a normal person, whether you're on a date at an ethnic restaurant or out for a work lunch at a hoagie shop.

The hardest—but best—part of this task? You're making the decisions. There is no gimmick here. We all have different taste buds, habits, and cravings. Different foods make us happy. The best I can do is clue you in to low-calorie foods generally regarded as awesome and warn you against the nonobvious pitfalls you'll encounter. Once you're armed with the right knowledge, you'll be wildly successful making your own decisions.

A Sense of Scale

One of your primary objectives during a day of dieting is to physically fill your belly to whatever extent you reasonably can. With that goal, it's actually sort of amazing how much foods can differ in their calories. Let's get a sense of scale by looking at three things you've likely consumed in the very same meal: wings, celery, and blue cheese dressing.

The dressing is the most caloric item on the plate. There are 150 calories in 2 tablespoons of Ken's Steak House Chunky Blue Cheese Dressing. If, for some disgusting reason, you wanted to subsist only on chunky blue cheese dressing for a day, you could take in 1,500 calories by eating only about 10 ounces of the stuff. If you were to sit down with the intent of consuming 10 ounces straight, chances are you'd get sick long before successfully doing so. But you'd also be amazed at how quickly you could absent-mindedly consume that much by plopping wings or spinach into the stuff. Imagine dipping a dozen wings into blue cheese dressing, slathering on a half ounce with each one. You'd quickly tack on about half your day's allotment of calories.

Let's move on to the wings. Turns out they've got a lot of calories, too. As anyone who's ever been to 10-cent Tuesday at a local wing joint can tell you, those things come in a wide variety of sizes. The little orange Godzillas they sell at Anchor Bar in Buffalo (the restaurant that invented the wing) could be close to 200 calories each. When national chains like Buffalo Wild Wings (a chain I'm embarrassed to admit originated a few miles from where I grew up) offer them at deep discounts, the shrimpy little suckers you get are more or less bones covered in skin and could be closer to 40. For the sake of simplicity, let's look at Pizza Hut, since their products tend to be fairly uniform.

There are about 660 calories in a twelve-piece order of Pizza Hut's traditional Buffalo wings. That's not great, obviously, but considering that there are 380 calories in a single slice of the Hut's large pepperoni pan pie, it's not so bad. Still, you're getting about 110 calories from two of them. Can you eat two and stop? That's impossible for most people, who are more likely to eat the entire dozen.

Now on to the celery. Actually, celery offers more bulk per calorie than you could consume in large quantities without overtaxing your digestive system. Contrary to popular belief, there aren't "negative" calories in the fibrous, faintly green stalks of *Apium graveolens,* but there are astonishingly few. You'd have to eat 700 grams of the stuff—a pound and a half, which is about one large head—to get 100 calories.

That's right, you could either eat two wings or a pound of celery for about 100 calories. Maybe that's what makes celery such a great companion to peanut butter and cheese, two of the most calorie-dense foods we have?

So here you have a sense of scale: One and a half tablespoons of blue cheese dressing, two wings, and a full pound of celery are caloric equals. Imagine these three things lined up next to one another on your kitchen counter and you'll understand why we're hunting for calorie bargains. Keep these examples in mind during our discussion of what to eat; while you'll lose weight by controlling your calories no matter what you eat, the types of foods you choose will make a huge difference in keeping you from getting too hungry while dieting.

Stuff You Can Nuke: Frozen Food

I heart my microwave. I don't care if that's cool or not, it's true. Maybe you'd prefer to avoid nuking any of the organic veggies you carefully selected at the farmer's market, but I find it hard to imagine life without my microwave. It is, quite simply, the best tool a dieter has.

Consider this: A year or so ago I read an article in the *Washington Post* about Ralph Friedgen, the football coach at the University of Maryland who lost 100 pounds eating food provided by a company called Medifast. The diet plan was suggested by a concerned alumnus who, as it happens, worked for Medifast, so the coach probably got some sort of discount, but I definitely got the impression this service was sort of expensive. I mentioned this to my mom, and she said one of her coworkers had similar success buying a week's allotment of frozen meals from some fancy company but gave up on her diet because it was too pricey.

"So, were these meals somehow special or, like, different from the ones at the grocery store?" I asked.

"No, I don't think so," she replied.

"Why the hell didn't she just go to the grocery store and buy the meals herself for $3 each instead of giving up her diet?" I asked.

There was no good answer. There never is.

Medifast sells oatmeal, soup, and diet shakes at a rate of something like $300 for a four-week supply. This deal appeals to some people. Friedgen told the *Post* he gave up on a previous diet because "it required him to shop for certain kinds of food" and this one didn't. I'm going to let you in on a little secret: If you venture into the frozen food aisle of the supermarket, you'll find that several companies sell prepared foods that are very similar to the stuff you buy from weight-loss companies at a fraction of the cost.

Single-serving microwave meals are such a great weight-loss tool that companies are apparently able to do little more than slip them into their own boxes and sell them to people who are too lazy to shop for themselves. That's pretty brilliant, actually. The simplest thing in the world—portion control—seems magical to some people. So it's easy for wily capitalists to profit from them.

Cooking is cool right now, so feel free to ignore this section if you're looking to get your Betty Crocker on every day, but I find microwave meals to be an excellent way to experience some of my favorite foods without the hassle of cooking or the expense of eating out. Plus, it takes about five minutes to make a meal and "do the dishes" (read: recycle the plastic tray) rather than an hour or more.

I'm not alone. According to a study by *Frozen Food Age* magazine—yes, such a publication exists—two thirds of shopping trips result in the purchase of frozen food. The biggest proportion of those sales comes from frozen dinners. Americans eat billions and billions of dollars' worth of these things every year, and 80 percent come from national brands you can find everywhere.

Stouffer's Lean Cuisine, Weight Watchers Smart Ones, and Healthy Choice are the sales titans in the mainstream market, while Amy's, Kashi, Eating Right, and Michelina's all have a niche.

People often ask me if I prefer one brand to another. I don't. In fact, I pretty much always buy whichever label is on sale (one always is), augmenting the weekly bargains with a few tried-and-true favorites from across the brand spectrum. I get around to all of them, too. Having eaten these things for a few years now, I'm always eager to try anything new or different. Every brand seems to do some things really well and other things very poorly, so there's no easy answer to "What kind should I buy?"

However, the stakes are pretty high. A frozen food flame-out really sucks. There are few things more frustrating than eagerly opening the microwave door only to discover a goopy, flavorless mess. Maybe you're the sort of person who can guiltlessly toss a bad meal out after a few bites and find something else. I, however, am not, so I've soldiered through some bad ones. I've put together these tips to save you either miserable meals or money. I've had nearly every type of low-cal frozen meal on the market, so consider these recommendations authoritative. Here are the best and worst by genre, with picks for each ordered from best to worst.

Pizza

AWESOME
Lean Cuisine Roasted Garlic Chicken Pizza—Wood Fire Style (330 calories)
They say: "Tender white meat chicken, roasted garlic, onions, and reduced-fat mozzarella cheese with a creamy garlic sauce on a crispy thin crust."
Chubster says: Everything from Lean Cuisine's pizza oven is pretty good, but this is the best. There is a strong garlic flavor, and the chicken and sauce both taste great. Perhaps the best part of the Lean Cuisine pizzas is that they come in three different kinds of crust. This is the medium thickness, but the Deep Dish Three Meat Pizza (390 calories) is a nice splurge, and the thinner Mushroom Pizza (300 calories) is excellent when you want to save a few calories.

Trader Joe's Reduced Guilt Pizza Primavera (250 calories)

They say: "Pizza Primavera with yellow squash, zucchini, eggplant, and bell peppers."

Chubster says: The crust on this puppy gets a little too crunchy for my taste, but the very impressive medley of flavors makes up for it. There's very little cheese on this pizza and no meat, which is how they keep the calories so low, but the generous serving of seasoned squash and red peppers makes it a great pick.

Eating Right Lean Pepperoni Thin Crust Pizza (360 calories)

They say: "Reduced-fat pepperoni and reduced-fat cheese on a brick oven crust."

Chubster says: I'm not sure if Eating Right's pizzas are actually that much better than their competitors' or if the brand's little flip-out foil box thingy just cooks them a lot better. The crust on this bad boy is always perfect. Eating Right is a Safeway brand (it's North America's third largest supermarket chain, behind SuperValu/Albertsons and Kroger/Ralph's/Frye's), but you can't get it some places. Sorry if you're missing out—maybe consider moving?

Michelina's Lean Gourmet Buffalo-Style Chicken Snack Rolls (380 calories for the whole package)

They say: "Spicy tomato sauce and white chicken in a light and flaky, fewer-calorie, golden crust. A newly inspired restaurant favorite."

Chubster says: These little devils aren't quite as light as I'd like, but when I have a craving for Buffalo wings and/or pizza rolls (which happens surprisingly often, considering I am not fifteen), they really hit the spot. Great flavor and the exact same nostalgically delicious crust you'd get from Totino's.

AWFUL

Smart Ones Four Cheese Pizza (370 calories)

They say: "Blend of reduced-fat mozzarella, Asiago, Parmesan, and Romano cheeses with a zesty tomato sauce on a stone-fired crust."

Chubster says: Smart Ones doesn't seem to do much in the pizza category, and this pie is evidence of why. It feels like a "token" offering from a company not willing to make the commitment to figuring out how to master the mysteries of the microwave and create a soft-yet-crispy pizza crust. This one is always crusty in the bad way. The cheese blend is decent, but the tomato sauce is not nearly as "zesty" as we might hope.

Michelina's Lean Gourmet Pepperoni Pizza (300 calories)

They say: "Light, flaky, and delicious pizza topped with a juicy tomato sauce, tasty pepperoni, and mozzarella cheese."

Chubster says: What sort of adjective is "juicy" applied to a pizza? If you're worried that means "soggy," you've smashed the nail on the head.

Kashi Thin Crust Pizza Margherita (260 calories)

They say: "Roma tomatoes, mozzarella, and provolone cheeses with a tomato-basil sauce on a wood-fired, thin crust made with Kashi 7 Whole Grains and Sesame and flax seed."

Chubster says: This tastes a lot more like a whole-wheat cracker than a pizza. The faint basil and tomato flavors are overwhelmed by the intensity of the dry, crunchy crust. It's a lot like eating a pile of autumn leaves with a dab of tomato sauce on them.

Other Italian

AWESOME

Lean Cuisine Chicken Carbonara (270 calories)

They say: "White meat chicken in a creamy parmesan sauce with turkey bacon, basil, and garlic over a bed of linguini."

Chubster says: That's turkey bacon? It sure tastes like real bacon to me! Carbonara is one of the heaviest traditional Italian dishes—the backbone of the authentic sauce is egg yolks, cured fatty pork, and a mix of dry cheeses—and this version manages to hit some of those same notes without all the calories. The sauce is also remarkably creamy for a light dinner.

Lean Cuisine Chicken Tuscan (280 calories)

They say: "Chicken tenderloins and linguine in a sun-dried tomato sauce served with broccoli and carrots."

Chubster says: Like all the choices in Lean Cuisine's line of slightly larger Dinnertime Selections, this is a very satisfying meal. The sun-dried tomatoes in the sauce actually taste like real sun-dried tomatoes, and the other veggies meld well under the sauce. The chicken isn't super tender, but it has decent flavor. The spices aren't particularly reminiscent of actual Italian food, however. LC's Jumbo Rigatoni with Meatballs is a lot closer to what you'd get in Campania, but at 400 calories, it makes for a pretty big calorie commitment for the day.

Smart Ones Chicken Parmesan (290 calories)

They say: "Seasoned chicken breast and spaghetti with marinara sauce topped with cheese."

Chubster says: The description is simple and so is the dish.

The marinara sauce, cheese, and noodles here are all decent, but the star of the show is a very nice cut of chicken breast. The red sauce has a nice bold flavor, and the cheese melts into a creamy pile.

AWFUL

Lean Cuisine Chicken with Lasagna Rollatini (290 calories)

They say: "Cheese lasagna rollatini with lightly breaded white meat chicken in a robust tomato sauce."

Chubster says: Rollatini isn't actually a type of pasta. It's not even an Italian word, but in the American version of Italian food it means something breaded and baked—which is just one indicator that this meal is going to go awry. The tomato sauce is anything but robust, and the cheese has a gummy consistency. The chicken slices have decent flavor but are oddly and unpleasantly thin.

Amy's Garden Vegetable Lasagna (290 calories)

They say: "Gluten-free tender rice noodles layered with creamy ricotta blended with a mixture of organic vegetables (spinach, zucchini, broccoli, carrots, and peas) and covered with a fresh-tasting tomato sauce."

Chubster says: At only 290 calories, this lasagna is one of the lightest ones you'll find. It tastes like it, too. Without meat *or* gluten, this thing is a sloppy, flavorless mess. The consistency of everything in the container is a little slimy, and the few little hints of flavor you find don't really go together. Also, whoever thought it was a good idea to put peas in lasagna clearly hasn't a drop of Italian blood in them. You might as well halve the little suckers and put them on a slice of pizza.

Lean Cuisine Chicken Club Panini (360 calories)
They say: "Grilled white meat chicken strips with crumbled bacon, tomatoes, cheese and ranch-style sauce on sourdough bread."
Chubster says: Almost all the Lean Cuisine "paninis" are pretty bad, but this one seems to be the worst. They're trying so damned hard to make something that tastes like it's bad for you (*yet it actually isn't—shhhhh!*), but they can't quite pull it off. Sorry, folks, but it's sort of impossible to get bacon and ranch sauce on two rather thick slices of bread in at 360 calories without making it gross. If something sounds too good to be true, it probably is. Look for meals that have a few intensely flavorful and high-cal ingredients combined with vegetables.

Eating Right Turkey Lasagna (370 calories)
They say: "Layers of pasta, tomato sauce, ground turkey, and vegetables topped with mozzarella cheese."
Chubster says: This might be the single worst frozen dinner on the market. I had it sitting in my freezer for a month before trying it; I should have waited longer. First, there's the unnatural smell that emanates from the oven while it cooks. It's pungent and gamey, and not in a good way. The flavor follows suit. And the consistency of the pasta and cheese is less than OK. All for just a hair less than 400 calories. There's nothing redeeming about this dish.

Other European

AWESOME
Eating Right Mediterranean Style Chicken with Linguini and Zucchini (230 calories)
They say: "We've combined tender white meat chicken with

tomatoes, yellow bell peppers, zucchini, and whole-wheat linguini, then topped it all off with a hearty, flavorful sauce."
Chubster says: I'm not sure this dish really exists out "in the
wild," but Eating Right's Med-style chicken has an excellent
flavor. It reminds me of the sort of thing you'd get at one of
those hippy-dippy restaurants that serves twelve kinds of
hummus but in a more reasonable portion.

Smart Ones Swedish Meatballs (270 calories)
They say: "Swedish Meatballs in a savory cream sauce with
wide pasta ribbons."
Chubster says: These are better than the Swedish meatballs
at Ikea. I'm sure that's a controversial statement, and I'm
no expert on Swedish meatballs (does anyone actually eat
them in some context besides an Ikea trip or in a microwave
meal?), but I really like these. The meat has great consistency, and the sauce is pleasantly creamy. I like to add a little
more pepper, but otherwise these are pretty great.

Lean Cuisine Stuffed Cabbage with Whipped Potatoes (210 calories)
They say: "Stuffed cabbage roll filled with a blend of beef and
pork, rice, and seasonings. Topped with a tomato sauce and
served with a side of whipped potatoes."
Chubster says: This is a healthy variation on a dish found in
most of northern and eastern Europe but chiefly associated
with Poles in the U.S. Many Americans have an odd aversion
to pickled cabbage—our ancestors found it a great way to get
vegetable vitamins during the cold winter months—so it's
not surprising that LC goes with a fresher, lighter variation
here. Happily they mix both beef and pork, which is the key
to getting that Old World flavor. I would prefer a sharper
flavor from the tomatoes, but it's still a nice option.

Lean Cuisine Steak Tips Dijon (280 calories)

They say: "Beef tips with roasted red skin potatoes and green beans."

Chubster says: It doesn't get any more classic than this—a little beef, a few potatoes, and some green beans. The appropriately salty brown sauce is what ties it all together, though.

AWFUL

Smart Ones Pasta Primavera (250 calories)

They say: "Tender bow tie pasta with broccoli florets and julienne-cut carrots in a creamy parmesan sauce."

Chubster says: There's nothing good about this meal. If you're going to make a primavera, it's essential you have crisp, fresh vegetables. The broccoli and carrots here don't qualify. The sauce isn't very cheesy, either, making for an incredibly bland dish.

Smart Ones Tuna Noodle Gratin (250 calories)

They say: "Tender chunks of tuna and linguini in a creamy sauce topped with toasted bread crumbs."

Chubster says: There's a good reason few microwave meals use tuna, and it has nothing to do with the meat being high in calories. It's generally hard to microwave fish and get something good out of it, and this meal proves the pitfalls: The tuna ends up slippery and tasteless. Neither the bread nor the sauce adds much, either.

Asian

AWESOME

Amy's Kitchen Indian Palak Paneer (300 calories)

They say: "Smooth, creamy palak paneer, made from organic spinach and soft Indian cheese, is lightly spiced with authentic Indian herbs and spices. Rajmah dal, made from organic red kidney beans in a ginger-garlic sauce and tender organic basmati rice complete this delicious meal."

Chubster says: This is the lightest of Amy's excellent Indian meals and also the best. I usually prefer Indian food with a lot more kick, but I understand it's impossible to sell microwave meals that are a 4 or 5 on the scale many restaurants use. Mattar Paneer (370 calories) and Paneer Tikka (320 calories) are traditionally pretty mild dishes anyway, so it's nice to switch things around and enjoy the creamy consistency of the spinach and cheese in Amy's version of the dish.

Trader Joe's Massaman Chicken (390 calories)
They say: "White chicken and vegetables with Massaman curry sauce over steamed rice."

Chubster says: The flavors here are right on—the vegetables and spices in this Massaman curry are straight-up carryout quality. However, at 390 calories it's not super light, and the 8-minute cooking time leaves a few pieces of the dark meat chicken too chewy. Still a quality option, though.

Eating Right Cashew Chicken (290 calories)
They say: "Your favorite flavors are all here: white meat chicken with sugar snap peas, shiitake mushrooms, red bell peppers, celery, carrots, bamboo shoots, cashew nuts and rice."

Chubster says: For some reason it seems really hard to seal mushroom flavor into a microwave meal. This dish does it. Sure, it's sort of generic, but the flavors are impressive, and the rice cooks up nice and fluffy.

Smart Ones Thai Style Chicken and Rice Noodles (260 calories)

They say: "Thai Style Chicken and Rice Noodles in a zesty peanut sauce."

Chubster says: Thai food is all the rage in Middle America right now, so the big boys have all rushed out to ape the Kashis and Amy's of the world with their own take on Thai. Mostly it just tastes like sweeter Chinese food. This dish is the exception—the peanut sauce is, indeed, zesty and will make you forget all about the takeout place down the street.

AWFUL

Kashi Sweet and Sour Chicken (320 calories)

They say: "Sliced chicken with roasted green beans and yellow pepper, red pepper, crimini mushrooms, onions, and edamame (soybeans), served over Kashi 7 Whole Grains Pilaf, and topped with a light, tangy sweet and sour sauce."

Chubster says: OK, so the meal isn't really bad, but it's nothing special, either. It's essentially the same thing you can get from the regular brands (substituting regular rice for pilaf) sold at twice the cost. Pass.

Smart Ones Orange Sesame Chicken (320 calories)

They say: "Breaded chicken tenderloins in a zesty sesame orange sauce with rice."

Chubster says: This is just one terrible meal from the godforsaken Fruit Inspirations line Smart Ones will hopefully be killing soon. Cloyingly sweet with no spicy counterbalance, the sauce tastes as though it was made from orange Tang.

Mexican

AWESOME

Kashi Mayan Harvest Bake (340 calories)

They say: "Plantains with roasted sweet potato, black beans, and kale. Spicy ancho sauce with pumpkin seed garnish served over Kashi seven whole grain polenta, plus amaranth."

Chubster says: Kashi's offerings are a little pricier than pretty much anything else out there, but you can see why with this dish. What other frozen dinners have plantains, kale, or polenta? Not all the Kashi dinners are worth the premium price and slightly higher calorie counts, but this one is. The textures are fantastic, and the variety of flavors is truly impressive.

Amy's Kitchen Black Bean Tamale Verde (330 calories)

They say: "All the ingredients for our Black Bean Tamales are carefully selected and prepared. The organic masa (ground and cooked corn) is poured onto individual parchments, filled with tender organic black beans and a mixture of organic vegetables, chilis and jalapenos, and then folded and steamed. The tamales are then unwrapped by hand, topped with our delicious verde sauce and served with a side of Spanish rice made from organic brown rice."

Chubster says: There are a lot of burritos and tamales on the market, but this one is tops. The black beans are wonderfully spiced, and it actually tastes like there are jalapeños and chilis in the sauce. The consistency of the masa dough is actually pretty similar to what you'd find in the husk at a Mexican restaurant, which is a miracle considering it's microwaved frozen food.

AWFUL

Amy's Southwestern Burrito (290 calories)

They say: "This burrito is made with fire-roasted poblano peppers, jalapeño peppers, black olives, and organic corn masa, combined with organic pinto beans and Monterey Jack cheese in an organic whole wheat tortilla."

Chubster says: This is a very good time to make an important point about Amy's, Kashi, and Trader Joe's. Which is that while they're lumped in with other "healthy" frozen meals, they're not really as light as many other options in the broad genre they're assigned to because of their emphasis on natural and organic ingredients. Actually, in terms of calories, they're a lot closer to traditional frozen meals than light ones, as you can see with this 5.5-ounce burrito that comes in at 290 calories. Others in the Amy's line are in the same range. This one is delicious and fairly satisfying, but for nearly 300 calories without a side, it's not much of a meal.

Smart Ones Chicken Enchiladas Suiza (290 calories)

They say: "Served in a zesty sour cream and green chile sauce with Spanish rice."

Chubster says: The tortillas always seem to be stiff and dry and the "green chile" blends with the sour cream to make one flavorless sludge.

Michelina's Lean Gourmet Santa Fe Style Rice and Beans (320 calories)

They say: "Santa Fe Style Rice and Beans in a Sour Cream and Mild Jalapeño Sauce. Seasoned rice with a delicious Tex-Mex blend of red and black beans topped with a mild Jalapeño sauce and cheddar cheese."

Chubster says: You can often find this meal for only $1, and it's almost worth that. "Mild" is a bit of an understatement to describe the sauce, which mostly tastes like warmed whole milk. The beans and rice have a nice consistency, though, so this isn't a bad companion to a single-serving burrito from Amy's (if you've got 600 calories for a meal) or doused in fresh salsa.

Comfort Food

AWESOME
Lean Cuisine Roasted Turkey Breast (290 calories)
They say: "Tender slices of roasted turkey tenderloins in a traditional gravy with stuffing, whipped potatoes, and green beans accented with cranberries."
Chubster says: This masterpiece might be my all-time favorite microwave meal. It's laid out in the package like an actual dinner would be on a plate, which makes me feel less like an unmarried man living alone in an apartment, and everything cooks perfectly. Thanksgiving-style turkey dinners are one of the original TV dinners, and it's clear that Stouffer's put its 70-plus years of experience into this meal. The turkey is incredibly flavorful, and the stuffing gets a nice little crust without going dry. Even the boring green beans are delicious thanks to a nice little kick from the cranberries.

Smart Ones Salisbury Steak (200 calories)
They say: "Salisbury Steak with a savory gravy and asparagus."
Chubster says: I'm not sure how ye olde Salisbury steak (invented by a Civil War veteran) came to be one of the most common microwave foods, but it is. This light version has all of the flavor you remember from your childhood when your mother was too sick or busy to cook—which is, of course, probably how the demand for frozen meals began. The onion-

flavored gravy is pretty decent, considering the process I imagine gravy goes through in order to win a place in a low-cal meal. There are versions of this with asparagus or macaroni and cheese; the mac 'n' cheese edition adds 80 calories and isn't as good.

Amy's Kitchen Chili and Cornbread Whole Meal (340 calories)

They say: "A soul-satisfying meal of cornbread and tasty organic chili with organic beans and vegetables and just enough spice to lift your spirits."

Chubster says: "Soul-satisfying" may be a bit of an overstatement, but this dish is, in fact, a hearty, home-style meal suitable for a fall Sunday. The chili has nice hot and sweet flavor—Amy's product developers apparently have a little more latitude with the spices than the more mainstream brands—and the cornbread is a really nice touch.

AWFUL

Lean Cuisine Salisbury Steak (260 calories)

They say: "Salisbury steak with macaroni and cheese."

Chubster says: Unlike the Smart Ones Salisbury Steak, this one *is* totally slimy—you can even see it from the way the gravy glistens in the photo on the front of the box. I realize that it sounds crazy to imply that this macaroni and cheese is much different from what you get in Lean Cuisine's standalone version, which is pretty good, but it seems that way to me. And, as I said, I eat enough of these things to notice the subtle differences.

Eating Right Baked Turkey (320 calories)

They say: "This is comfort food with a healthier twist. We've paired oven-roasted turkey and gravy with carrots and corn-

bread croutons, just the way you would if you had the time."
Chubster says: This meal isn't that terrible, but it stacks up poorly against the other turkey meals out there. I'm not sure how it can have so many calories compared to the mammoth Lean Cuisine version that has so much more food and flavor.

Michelina's Lean Gourmet Beef Pepper Steak and Rice (260 calories)

They say: "Beef pepper steak and rice with green peppers and onions, savory strips of seasoned beef in a light tomato sauce with fresh onions, and green peppers served over a bed of tender white rice."
Chubster says: As you can see from the description, there's a lot going on in this meal. Unfortunately, none of it is going very well. There's no dominant flavor here, which makes this meal less than satisfying—you'll forgot you ate it within a few minutes.

Satisfying a Sweet Tooth: Low-Cal Desserts

What do dieters eat for dessert? Believe it or not, you've got lots of great options. Cheesecake, tiramisu, and Chunky Monkey are obviously out. It's probably safest to avoid restaurant desserts altogether, since they're nearly always designed to be decadent. You should also forget about so-called healthier options like oatmeal cookies, which fall under the Bagel Paradox: The cookie recipe on the Quaker Oats container renders 140-calorie cookies that are pretty small. On that note, I'm also not usually a fan of the lighter versions of regular cookies and desserts you'll find at the store—Snack Wells, for example—which tend to be either nothing like the original or not significantly less caloric. Here's what to look for instead:

Fresh Fruit: You've probably heard this before, but fresh fruit really is your best dessert option on a diet. If you don't have a taste for the natural sweetness of grapes, cherries, oranges, and strawberries, now is a pretty good time to develop one. It won't be hard, trust me; it's just a matter of learning to appreciate a more subtle sweetness.

The dietary benefits are staggering, though. A whole pound of unpitted cherries—for me this is one serving; I love them—is only 290 calories. You could be a little more moderate about it and have a nice 150-calorie after-dinner snack. There are only about 2 calories in each medium-sized grape, meaning an entire cup is only about 100 calories.

An entire pound of strawberries is only about 150 calories. If you want to turn them into something a little fancier, the

---

☕ An Open Letter to the Folks Down at the Farmer's Market

I know some angry and disappointed hipsters are reading this book and wishing it were promoting organic vegetables, slow food, local produce, and the other big foodie trends of the moment. Perhaps it seems very unhip to be advocating the consumption of factory-farmed foods that are processed, frozen, and shipped across the country. I can only imagine what some crunchier hipsters think when I suggest purchasing food from Ronald McSatan himself instead of from some chick who uses baking soda as a deodorant. Sorry.

If you're not feeling my suggestions, you should instead check out Michael Pollan's *The Omnivore's Dilemma*. It will tell you a lot about how to hunt a feral pig in northern California but very little about how to lose weight, which is our primary objective here. Maybe Pollan's credo—"Eat food. Not too much. Mostly plants" and avoiding anything his grandmother would not have recognized as food—would be traditional accompaniment, angel food cake and whipped cream, can also be pretty light. One serving of regular angel food cake is only about 70 calories, while sugar-free whipped cream is only 20 calories per quarter cup. Combine them and, voilà, you have a superlight strawberry shortcake.

Ice Cream: Ice cream is my second favorite food after pizza, and I eat it pretty much every single day. How is that possible? I go with the light options from brands like Skinny Cow (a single serving cup of Dulce de Leche, 150 calories) or Breyer's (Chocolate Chip Cookie Dough sandwich, 160 calories) or a 150-calorie McDonald's cone. Look around, and you'll find a sugar-free or low-fat version of any flavor you like.

---

an effective weight-loss plan, but I haven't heard of anyone succeeding that way. Instead, Chubster is all about taking advantage of every modern convenience afforded us. In my unapologetically innovationist view, technology got us into this mess by making it possible to consume so many cheap calories while being so sedentary, and it'll somehow get us out of it, too.

I have very little interest in killing any animal myself or getting up early on Saturday morning to schlep down to a parking lot and pick out vegetables I can purchase for a similar price at a nearby grocery store, even if they do have the best arugula ever. Sorry, but that's just not my scene. Maybe people like Pollan are right that the stuff we eat today isn't even "food" and that it'll eventually poison us; however, life expectancy seems to be on an upward trajectory even if the light sour cream we now eat doesn't fit an organic dairy farmer's definition. Maybe I'll be proven a fool, but I'm putting my faith in common sense and scientific ingenuity.

Frozen Yogurt: Maybe it's a stretch to say I eat ice cream every day—sometimes I have frozen yogurt instead. Yogurt tends to be a little lighter than ice cream if you buy it at the grocery store, but there are, oddly, not as many single-serving options. You need to be very careful controlling your portions with a half-gallon—I think it's safer to stick with individually packaged portions, even at a much higher cost. I'm also a huge fan of the new pour-it-yourself places like Yogurtland and Pinkberry, where you can get exactly as much as you want and you know how much you took because you pay by the ounce. There are 18 calories per ounce in Yogurtland's basic tart vanilla flavor, and they have a nice selection of fresh fruit to top it with. Just steer clear of the chocolaty goodness next to the chopped-up bananas and raspberries. To figure calories, play it safe and just multiply the number of ounces you pay for by 20 for vanilla, adjusting accordingly if you go with a higher-calorie flavor like chocolate.

Fudgesicles: Fudgesicles—those vaguely cocoa-flavored frozen treats you remember from childhood—are also very diet-friendly. Popsicle brand makes them in a range of sizes with a variety of sweeteners—some have as few as 40 calories per bar. Other brands have similar options and calorie counts.

Popsicles: Popsicles are another almost-doesn't-need-to-be-counted dessert. (Note "almost.") Even an old-fashioned Firecracker is only 35 calories and a sugar-free Popsicle-brand popsicle is only about 15. Crystal Light's frozen treats, which come in flavors like Cherry Pomegranate, Lemonade, and Wild Strawberry, are even tastier and also only 15 calories.

Meringues: Meringues, a French dessert made with sugar and egg whites, is a decadent but light treat, especially in dried and unadorned cookie form. Cookies are generally a high-calorie indulgence, but meringue cookies—I've seen Miss Meringue brand, which makes 10-calorie mini meringues, popping up in grocery stores lately—are a notable exception.

Rice Cakes: Rice cakes are an amazing diet food because they're so adaptable—they make for a great snack with either savory or sweet seasonings. The Quaker Quakes line has some of the better options on the market, including flavors like Apple Cinnamon, Caramel Corn, and Vanilla Crème Brule. The Apple Cinnamon is particularly good and tastes a lot like an apple pie. Eight of the tiny cakes have only 60 calories, and the variety of flavors can satisfy a wide range of cravings that are hard to satisfy healthfully.

Stuff You Can Get at the Drive-Through: Fast Food

Remember when you first heard about the Taco Bell Drive-Thru Diet? It seemed like a joke, right? *Ha-ha-ha! Healthy fast food! What an oxymoron! Losing weight while eating drive-through food! OMG! Stupid fat Americans!*

Actually, it isn't as much of a joke as people think. You can absolutely lose weight eating nothing but fast food if you want to. In fact, while fast-food chains are justifiably maligned for dumbing down American cuisine and giving people a taste for things that are fast, cheap, and fatty, most are also surprisingly friendly to dieters. Sure, they have triple bacon cheeseburgers on the menu—and they'd probably give one to your five-year-old along with a Disney toy if you ask nicely—but, as a rule, they're all about options, and if you want something healthy, you can get it.

In fact, after Morgan Spurlock did his hatchet job on Mickey D's, a guy named Chris Coleson set the record straight. You've probably never heard of Coleson because his experience doesn't fit with the convenient anti–fast-food narrative you've been fed for decades.

Maybe this isn't the sort of thing you want to read in a

🍔 Question: How accurate are restaurant and packaged food calorie counts?

Answer: Not very.

A 2010 study found that published restaurant calorie counts are 18 percent below what they should be on average, and the nutrition labels on frozen foods are 8 percent below. The project started when a nutrition professor at Tufts University noticed she wasn't losing weight the way she should have been and decided to toss a few dozen labeled foodstuffs in a calorimeter to see how they actually burned up. The results were published in the *Journal of the American Dietetic Association.*

This is a little heartbreaking, I know. It seems totally unfair that while you're relying on this information to make a huge life change, it might very well be flawed. Yet it's the best we have.

A few things to consider:

• Researchers may have picked items they suspected were inaccurately labeled, making the problem seem worse than it is. The study says it used typical American foods diet book, but the Academy Award–nominated documentary *Super Size Me* is complete bullshit. During his "experiment," Spurlock force-fed himself the unhealthiest food he could find on the McDonald's menu. In fact, he ate the equivalent of 9.26 Big Macs a day! No one does that unless they're trying to make themselves sick on camera to fleece a bunch of yuppies out of $9 for a ticket to a movie that does little more than reinforce their bourgeois bigotry by depicting the foods accessible to members of lower socioeconomic classes as

that were supposed to be less than 500 calories per serving and among those with the fewest calories on a restaurant's menu. But it wasn't a randomized sampling of those foods—it's whatever foods they picked.

• The Food and Drug Administration actually spots food sellers a 20 percent margin of error, so many of these mistakes wouldn't even be corrected by the government. That margin seems pretty generous to me, and it could actually influence the success of your diet, since that's quite possibly about what you're cutting. What can you do about this? Not much besides writing your congressman.

• It's often easy to tell when you're getting a slightly larger portion than might be officially counted. For example, McDonald's soft serve cones are supposed to be 150 calories, but most employees are a little more generous than that. I count the smallest cone I've ever gotten as 150 and adjust up toward 250 when they top off that small with a little extra goodness. Use common sense when something seems a little too good to be true.

somehow inferior to the equally unhealthy restaurant foods they enjoy. The movie *is* incredibly disgusting—just not the way Spurlock and his fans think. A film called *Venti Size Me* probably wouldn't make as much money since it doesn't repeat misinformation about why Americans are fat, but I'm absolutely positive I could duplicate Spurlock's experience with a yuppie-friendly chain like Starbucks or Panera Bread and make myself *at least* as fat as he did.

Coleson, on the other hand, lost 80 pounds in six months eating two McDonald's meals every day. The then forty-two-year-old Virginia man did it by ordering salads (hey, Morgan, they have salads at McDonald's!) along with normal-size hamburgers, apple dippers, wraps, and the like. Yes, all these things exist on the McDonald's menu, and, no, they're not disgusting. Coleson, as best I can tell, did this, not as a political statement or to gain money and fame, but because he genuinely appreciated the excellent experience and impressive value McDonald's offers customers. As do I.

People bash McDonald's, but they're the motherfucking Gandhi of chain restaurants compared to the Cheesecake Factory. Now, taking the Cheesecake Factory back to the woodshed is the bread and butter of the Eat This, Not That series (*Men's Health* editor David Zinczenko, who writes those books, is obsessive in his hatred of the place—I suspect he's got an evil ex who's a waitress there), so I won't rehash all that, but it's absolutely true that they sell salads with close to 2,000 calories in them and you should avoid eating there on the Chubster diet.

Of course, there were probably a few people who ate at a Cheesecake Factory in an upscale mall before waddling to the theater next door to watch *Super Size Me* and look down their noses at the offerings of the ultimate American common man's restaurant.

The point is that fast food isn't evil. Like pretty much any-thing else, it offers good and bad choices for dieters. You need to know what the smart choices are, then order accordingly.

Here's a breakdown of what to get at our nation's top ten fast-food chains according to their sales rankings from *QSR* magazine, the definitive source of all things related to the Quick Service Restaurant industry, along with a few hipster-friendly wildcards. The goal here is to find foods that are deli-cious and filling but don't blow your caloric budget for the day.

For each spot there's a smart pick, a stupid pick, and a borderline indulgence. Those categories are all relative, de-pending greatly on the restaurant in question. That is, even the dumbest decision at Subway (a 6-inch meatball mari-nara sub with bacon and mayonnaise, 715 calories) might be better than the smart pick at a place like Five Guys. Some of these places are going to be rough even with the smartest pick and are best reserved for special occasions. We're just trying to arm you with information to navigate the menu wherever you are.

MCDONALD'S
Keep in Mind: The best choices tend to be grilled chicken dishes, so aim for those. Remember that a few fries won't set you back too far, but you need to eat them one at a time because those calories add up quickly. Avoid most of the beef—it's not marked by a great flavor-to-calorie ratio, as you probably already know.

The Best and Most Responsible Choice: Honey Mustard Snack Wrap with Grilled Chicken (230 calories) plus a side salad with Newman's Own Low Fat Balsamic Vinaigrette (60 calories for both) or Premium Bacon Ranch Salad with Grilled Chicken (260 calories) and get the balsamic dressing. If you want dessert, go for a small ice cream cone (150 calories).

A Minor Indulgence: A six-piece Chicken McNuggets (280 calories without sauce—add 60 calories per pack for sauce) and small French fries (230 calories).

Dear God, No: The ever-elusive McRib (500 calories) is bad, but worry more about the deceptively benign-sounding Premium Crispy Chicken Club Sandwich (630 calories) or a large French fry (500 calories).

SUBWAY

Keep in Mind: Subway is well established as "The Healthy Fast Food brand." Thanks, Jared! Mostly, that reputation matches their menu, but watch out for cheese (40 calories per package), which is included in a sandwich's price but not in the calorie total printed on the napkins. Add all the veggies they'll give you—stare at the Sandwich Artists intently and/or ask nicely if they're skimping on something and they'll normally hook you up unless a manager just lectured them about the cost of olives. Also keep in mind that Subway's wheat bread is not really all that wheaty and differs only trivially in calories, so unless you actually like wheat bread better (I do), just get the white bread. Oh, and avoid the sauces like the plague—you could easily end up with a normal 6-inch sub's worth of calories in Chipotle Ranch dressing added to your sandwich. And keep your damned hands away from the cookie case. Seriously, with more than 200 calories each, those things are bad news.

The Best and Most Responsible Choice: 6-inch Oven Roasted Chicken Breast with all the veggies and no cheese (320 calories) plus apple slices (35 calories) or chicken noodle soup (80 calories).

A Minor Indulgence: 6-inch BLT with light mayo (410 calories) or a foot-long Turkey Breast (570 calories), which is a whole lot of food.

Dear God, No: 6-inch Chicken and Bacon Ranch (570 calories) or 6-inch Cold Cut Combo with mayonnaise (520 calories).

BURGER KING

Keep in Mind: Burger King is not doing very well at the moment. If you ask me, the restaurant's lackluster options for health-conscious consumers are part of the problem. The King's men are still trying to break away from the sad era when they were apparently trying to be a poor man's Carl's Jr., and their sales have been weak as they cater to "Super Fans" (read: young, fat, nerdy males who eat there several times a week) and drag their feet on updating a menu that looks like what their top competitors were doing during the middle of the Bush administration. I would say you should avoid the restaurant like the plague, but, if you have occasion to go there, stop by while you still can—it likely won't be around in a decade.

The Best and Most Responsible Choice: Burger King's menu is an absolute mess; there aren't many Chubster-friendly items here. The five-piece Crown-Shaped Chicken Tenders (230 calories) and the BK Veggie Burger (400 calories) both qualify. Why does anyone want to eat chicken shaped like a crown? How many fast-food customers want a veggie burger? Don't fall back on the Side Garden Salad—Burger King's somehow has 330 calories in it. How? Who the fuck knows with this place! Just use 10 extra calories and get a small fry (340 calories).

A Minor Indulgence: The Tendergrill Chicken Sandwich (470 calories), which you may remember as the BK Broiler or one of the other five names they've tried to give that thing, is relatively tasty. Maybe just save some cash (and calories) and get the "Buck Double" $1 double cheeseburger or a Whopper Jr. (440 calories each). Actually, maybe ordering the Hershey's Sundae Pie (310 calories) isn't a bad idea, either—it's one of the best fast-food desserts available anywhere and certainly one of the few truly stellar items on Burger's King's sad little menu.

Dear God, No: Tendercrisp Garden Salad (670 calories) is so ridiculous, it almost makes a Steakhouse XT Burger Value Meal (1,500 calories with medium fries and regular Coca-Cola) seem like a rational choice.

STARBUCKS

Keep in Mind: Plain old coffee is extremely diet-friendly; most other items at Starbucks are not. Like those "Bread" places (Panera, Wildflower, Atlanta, Paradise) that serve hearty sandwiches with semi-exotic ingredients, Starbucks lulls people into a false sense of diet security with soft earth tones and world music. Drink the coffee; steer clear of the cookies, cakes, and especially enticing seasonal coffee drinks that are more like milk shakes than coffee.

The Best and Most Responsible Choice: Coffee, espresso, and tea are all pretty much calorie-free. Be careful what you add, though, because enough half-and-half to lighten it up and two packets of sugar change the game (74 calories). Likewise, if you want to add honey to your tea, you're going to need to log it (64 calories per tablespoon). The Chicken on Flatbread with Hummus Artisan Snack Plate (250 calories) is the only food I can recommend in good conscience.

A Minor Indulgence: A Grande Caffe Latte with nonfat milk (170 calories). If you have to have something sweet, look for anything with "mini" in the name or the Marshmallow Dream Bar (210 calories). A scone (400 calories and up, depending on the flavor) with black coffee is also an option since the total calories for the drink and pastry aren't too bad.

Dear God, No: Peppermint White Chocolate Mocha (470 calories) or a Venti Chai Latte, which is very heavy for a drink, especially if you get it with whole milk (398 calories). Also avoid foods like Banana Nut Loaf (490 calories).

WENDY'S

Keep in Mind: Wendy's Old Fashioned Hamburgers is the official name of this burger joint, and much of the menu is, indeed, old-fashioned. That doesn't mean it's bad. Though they seem to vary their lineup of salads every year or so without great results, there are some stellar and totally unique options here. Where else can you get chili at a drive-through?

The Best and Most Responsible Choice: The sour cream and chive baked potato (320 calories) and small chili (220 calories) make an excellent pair. The broccoli and cheese baked potato (330 calories) is also good.

A Minor Indulgence: Homestyle Chicken Go Wrap (320 calories), a Caesar side salad (250 calories), and a Junior Frosty (150 calories).

Dear God, No: Avoid the salads. The BLT Cobb Salad (670 calories) and Apple Pecan Chicken Salad (580 calories) are both pretty poor compared to the offerings at other fast-food joints.

TACO BELL

Keep in Mind: Taco Bell is the top outlet in the Yum! Brands gang that also gives us KFC, Pizza Hut, Long John Silver's, and A&W restaurants. History lesson: Basically, these places exist only because no reputable fast-food joint would serve Pepsi in the good ol' days and the soft drink maker needed to sell cheap sugar water to burger-eaters somehow. The entire Yum! chain is pretty shoddy—mostly the restaurants just want to trick people into trying "new" products with intense advertising for gimmicky menu items that are essentially slight variants of other dishes. And they're not very diet-friendly, either.

The Best and Most Responsible Choice: Two Fresco Crunchy Tacos (150 calories each) and an order of Mexican Rice (130 calories).

A Minor Indulgence: Fresco Bean Burrito (350 calories) or the half-pound Combo Burrito (460 calories), which are a little higher in calories than you'd like but will at least fill you up.

Dear God, No: The light-sounding Chicken Ranch Taco Salad (910 calories) makes a Nachos BellGrande (770 calories) look like a good option.

PIZZA HUT

Keep in Mind: Pizza is generally not a light food and Pizza Hut doesn't sell it in convenient single slices, which makes this restaurant of little use to a dieter.

The Best and Most Responsible Choice: The new Fit 'N Delicious Pizzas are the company's attempt to healthify their menu. How are they? Meh. The lowest-cal options (Diced Red Tomato, Mushroom, and Jalapeño; Green Pepper, Red Onion, and Diced Red Tomato) still have 150 calories per slice. The Baked Hot Wings are only about 50 calories each, so they can be good, too.

A Minor Indulgence: The Medium Thin 'N Crispy Pizza with pepperoni on it has about 200 calories per slice, so you could split the pizza with another person without things getting too far out of control (800 calories for half the pie). Add

50 calories per slice if you want the traditional pan version (I would). The 6-inch Personal Pan Pizza is an easier way to control portions—the cheese version has 590 calories but add only 20 calories more for pepperoni.

Dear God, No: A single slice of the large Stuffed Crust Meat Lover's has 480 calories in it. The 9-inch Personal PANormous Pizza is marketed as a single-serving pizza, but it's 1,100 calories with just cheese.

DUNKIN' DONUTS

Keep in Mind: Dunkin' Donuts is known for selling, *mmmm-mmmm,* doughnuts. So, yeah, it's not the healthiest spot in town. They're trying, though.

The Best and Most Responsible Choice: The Egg White Turkey Sausage Flatbread (290 calories) is a treat. The Egg and Cheese Wake-Up Wrap (180 calories) is another great option. Don't forget the coffee—it's filling and totally calorie-free so long as it's black. If you want something a little milder, you can get a small coffee with skim milk for only 15 calories.

A Minor Indulgence: Despite the fact that it's on their diet-centric "DD Smart" menu, the ham, egg, and cheese muffin is 360 calories. That's a little silly considering that the McDonald's menu item it's directly ripping off—the vaunted Egg McMuffin—is only 300 calories. I'd rather have the chain's authentic Boston Kreme Donut, which is 310 calories, and a giant black coffee.

Dear God, No: The multigrain bagel is on the "DD Smart" menu, but it has 390 calories plain. Is a dry multigrain bagel really what you want for almost 400 calories? I doubt it. That's the same as their éclair, and it isn't anywhere near as delicious.

KFC

Keep in Mind: Fried chicken is not healthy. Grilled chicken, however, can be. KFC sells grilled chicken—and some nice home-style sides—which can make for a nice meal so long as you steer clear of the fried temptations, not to mention the biscuits (180 calories each).

The Best and Most Responsible Choice: The salads are good options, provided you choose your dressing carefully. The Grilled Chicken Caesar Salad is only 210 calories—without dressing or croutons. The croutons add 70 calories and the Buttermilk Ranch dressing, 160 calories. The Marzetti Light Italian dressing, on the other hand, has only 15 calories per serving. Several traditional sides, like green beans (20 calories), mashed potatoes with gravy (120 calories), three-bean salad (70 calories), and corn on the cob (140 for the full ear) are also nice options. Add a grilled chicken breast (210 calories) to those and you've got yourself a nice little meal that's very satisfying.

A Minor Indulgence: The Original Recipe chicken breast has only 150 calories without skin or breading. If you can manage to contain yourself to a few nibbles of the delicious fried skin, you can get the old-timey flavor for only about 200 calories.

Dear God, No: The KFC Famous Bowls Mashed Potato with Gravy (700 calories) makes an Original Recipe chicken breast (320 calories) and a few low-cal sides look like a decent option. I won't even address the Double Down in the hope it's already off the menu by the time you read this.

SONIC DRIVE-IN

Keep in Mind: Ah, Sonic, the bastion of all things Americana. Some locations even have carhops who still wear roller skates! Considering the place is so steadfastly old-fashioned, you might expect it to be a wasteland for dieters, but, happily, it isn't.

The Best and Most Responsible Choice: The grilled chicken salad (250 calories) ain't nothin' special, but she'll do. Be careful about adding the so-called light ranch dressing (110 calories) and instead go with the fat-free Italian (40 calories). If you want something fried on the side, go with the tots (200 calories for a medium) over the fries (330 calories for the medium) or any of the other oddities on the menu (310-calorie Pickle-O's).

A Minor Indulgence: A Sonic corn dog mysteriously and miraculously has only 210 calories in it. The old standby Sonic Burger isn't great on its own (560 calories), but it's easy to dress it up with jalapeños, grilled onions, green chilies, and the like for only a few calories more. That's a pretty big indulgence, sure, but if you're craving a good old-fashioned slab of Sonic's beef, it will hit the spot.

Dear God, No: Where to begin? The foot-long Coney (710 calories) and a large onion rings (640 calories) would leave you eating nothing but salad the rest of the day. A Frito chili pie (940 calories for the large, 490 for the medium) is crazy high in calories considering it is, ostensibly, composed largely of tomatoes and corn. I'm conveniently ignoring the fact that nearly half the menu is made up of desserts and drinks and they're pretty much all terrible for you, so steer clear of those and go with the easy, smart, and delicious Chubster-friendly choices outlined above.

CHIPOTLE

Keep in Mind: Chipotle has a limited menu, and most items come in huge portions. Also, a lot of the ingredients on the counter tend to be pretty high in calories. Try to get your flavors from the salsas—they'll give you all three types of tomato salsa on the same burrito without charge if you ask nicely—and avoid the cheese, sour cream, and guacamole. Also keep in mind that a bag of those lime-tinged chips has 570 calories in it.

The Best and Most Responsible Choice: A burrito bowl with chicken, rice, beans, and salsa (520 calories).

A Minor Indulgence: A carnitas burrito with all three kinds of salsa, lettuce, and cheese (660 calories).

Dear God, No: The regular burrito with steak, rice, beans, corn, cheese, sour cream, and guacamole (1,200 calories). And that's without the chips.

PANDA EXPRESS

Keep in Mind: Panda has very, very smart and very, very stupid choices sitting right next to one another in the warming trays. It's important to look up the nutrition information for whatever you order, because you could easily triple your calorie counts with bad choices.

The Best and Most Responsible Choice: The two-item meal with Broccoli Beef (130 calories) and Mushroom Chicken (220 calories) and a side of mixed veggies (70 calories).

A Minor Indulgence: The two-item meal with Broccoli Chicken (180 calories) and Mongolian Beef (200 calories) and a side of veggie spring rolls (160 calories).

Dear God, No: The three-item meal with Beijing Beef (690 calories), Honey Walnut Shrimp (370 calories), and Orange Chicken (400 calories) and a side of fried rice (570 calories).

FIVE GUYS

Keep in Mind: Five Guys is one of those places a lot of people like because it's a hip and fashionable fast-food experience. It's amazing how eager upper-middle-class Americans are to drink up the "anything old-fashioned is good" Kool-Aid and eat someplace with a red-and-white checkerboard motif even if it's selling some of the biggest and greasiest meals around. Even President Obama likes this place. However, the Virginia chain's food is extremely unhealthy, and I'd never waste the calories on it.

The Best and Most Responsible Choice: The "Little" hamburger starts off at 480 calories, bare-ass naked. The "Regular" cheeseburger, on the other hand, is 840 calories, which is about what you'd find in *two* McDonald's Double Cheeseburgers. How is Obama able to stay so much slimmer than Big Mac–lovin' Bill Clinton? Must be all that basketball. So what is the best and most responsible choice? Let's go with the veggie sandwich—at 440 calories, it's a tiny bit lighter than a Wendy's quarter-pound single (470 calories), but at least it's, *ummm,* vegetarian.

A Minor Indulgence: Did I mention you can't even get a single-size portion of french fries here? The 310-calorie "single serving" listed in their nutrition information is actually just half a 620-calorie regular serving! Disgusting. As for a minor indulgence, try ordering a big bag of sliced pickles (10 calories for a dozen) and telling the dude behind the counter you'll make a mess with the damn peanuts unless he hooks you up.

Dear God, No: The bacon cheeseburger with mayonnaise and BBQ sauce (1,080 calories) plus a large fry (1,464 calories).

CHICK-FIL-A

Keep in Mind: Most people who go into Chick-fil-A get fried chicken, but that's not all that's available. In fact, you can get a grilled version of almost anything your friends order fried, and their salads are pretty impressive. Just avoid the little extras—sauces and the like—they make it so easy to add on.

The Best and Most Responsible Choice: The Chick-fil-A Chargrilled and Fruit Salad (230 calories) is a great pick even if you add croutons (60 calories) and the Fat-Free Honey Mustard dressing (60 calories). To keep it super light, go without the bits of baked bread and choose the very vinegary Light Italian dressing (15 calories).

A Minor Indulgence: The Chick-fil-A Chargrilled Chicken Sandwich (300 calories) is a nice pick—just make sure you don't mistakenly order the Club version, which adds 110 calories. You can do a small waffle fry (310 calories) too, so long as you can summon the strength not to bump that up to a medium or add cheese for dipping.

Dear God, No: The regular fried chicken sandwich (400 calories) and the deluxe version thereof (490 calories) are both bad picks, but getting four fried Chick-n-strips (500 calories) is the worst thing you can do. Also avoid dipping anything in ranch sauce (100 calories for ¾ ounce) or getting one of their fancy milk shakes (930 calories for the Peppermint Chocolate Chip).

JASON'S DELI

Keep in Mind: There is a common misconception that all deli sandwiches are as diet-friendly as Subway's. Nope. I won't even try to discuss Quiznos (ugh), which has very little to offer dieters, but since the rapidly expanding Texas brand Jason's Deli calls itself healthy ("At Jason's Deli, we're all about healthy food"), they're worth examining.

The Best and Most Responsible Choice: The Mediterranean Wrap (320 calories) is the lightest thing on the menu—and it's not that light. Get that and the Fresh Fruit Cup without dip (90 calories) and get out of this place thanking your lucky stars you didn't fall into something awful.

A Minor Indulgence: I'm a sucker for a Reuben, and I love turkey pastrami and corned turkey almost as much as the real stuff, so it's hard to pass on the Turkey Reuben (510 calories). At more than 500 calories, though, it's a little silly to have it on the "A Little Lighter Menu." Well, maybe not . . .

Dear God, No: The Nutty Mixed Up Salad (920 calories) is bad news. So is the Big Chef Salad (500 calories without dressing). But it's the Taco Salad with Southwest Chicken Chili (1,907 calories) that really exposes Jason's as not quite as Jaredesque as their marketing suggests. That's a salad with chicken chili that's about a day's worth of calories for most people? Places that are "all about healthy food" don't lay traps for people with 1,900-calorie salads. Salad, chicken, and chili should be safe words for dieters—it's a shame they aren't at Jason's.

EL POLLO LOCO

Keep in Mind: Believe it or not, El Pollo Loco is now the nation's thirty-fifth largest fast-food chain, ranked above better-known brands like Baskin-Robbins, Boston Market, In-N-Out, and Sbarro. This humble OC-based chain earned it, too. It's a great spot for calorie counters, with a menu based mostly on grilled chicken (they'll even take the skin off for you!) with lots of options involving veggies and a killer salsa bar.

The Best and Most Responsible Choice: The skinless grilled chicken breast (180 calories) with mashed potatoes and gravy (120 calories) and a small side salad with Light Creamy Cilantro Dressing (140 calories total).

A Minor Indulgence: The Sirloin Steak Chili (160 calories for small, 430 for large) and a Taco al Carbón (160 calories).

Dear God, No: The Twice Grilled Burrito (800 calories)

with a Chicken Tostada Salad (900 calories) topped with regular Creamy Cilantro Dressing (190 calories).

WHITE CASTLE

Keep in Mind: Harold and Kumar only cemented what those in the know already understood: There's no such thing as "too far" to drive to White Castle. For dieters, this is both a wonderful and a terrible place. Terrible because most of the menu items are relatively unhealthy. Wonderful because the portions are small enough for you to sample the forbidden without making a huge calorie commitment. Still, White Castle should not be a regular stop on the Chubster diet. If you do happen to be here, don't order anything in the "sack" size. Also, don't order any of the chicken or fish. Counterintuitively, their fried fish and fried chicken are the most caloric things on the menu, with the fish and chicken ring sliders having more than double the calories of the beef burger.

The Best and Most Responsible Choice: Two Original Sliders (140 calories each) and a Saver-size fry (350 calories).

A Minor Indulgence: A Double Cheeseburger Slider (300 calories) and a Saver-size Sweet Potato fry (420 calories).

Dear God, No: A sack of Fish Nibblers (1,100 calories) and five mozzarella sticks (500 calories).

▦ Common Conversions

1 ounce = 28 grams
1 ounce = 2 tablespoons
1 ounce = 6 teaspoons
1 cup = 8 fluid ounces
1 pound = 16 ounces

Stuff That Scares Your Aunt: Ethnic Food

What wat do you order at an Ethiopian restaurant? Are you better off ordering the naan or the rice with your Indian curry? These are tough questions, to be sure. Weight-loss books usually steer clear of ethnic cuisine for good reason: It's really tough to figure out what's in front of you.

Most of the best ethnic restaurants are not part of chains large enough to publish nutrition information. And even some of the ones that are part of chains don't offer such info. This makes things a bit of a crapshoot.

Even if I tell you definitively what's in the dishes at any one hole-in-the-wall ethnic joint, the only way to get the information from the hidden gems in your city is either to ask the chef (he or she might tell you if you're a loyal customer) or have them tested by a calorimeter. Considering the cheapest calorimeter I can find on Google Shopping is $11,462 and most nutrition labs aren't gonna do you a solid, that's out of the question.   Yet, you're probably going to eat ethnic food during this diet, and you need to know how to count those calories. So we're going to do our best—counting up the calories in the ingredients from available recipes, comparing local restaurants to published information from national chains, and using a little common sense. Chances are, you can taste anything that adds a nontrivial number of calories (it's not hard to tell when a bunch of butter or cream has been added to something), so make sure you're keeping it real with yourself. After that, order carefully and hope for the best. Here are picks for various types of ethnic food, based on the total number of calories in each dish and how filling it is. The lowest calorie counts aren't always the smartest pick—ubiquity and predictability also come into play here, meaning that unless you're ordering the item at the specific restaurant mentioned here, you probably want to play it safe and order something that's consistently light wherever you order it.

ITALIAN

Keep in Mind: Italian food can be great or terrible for dieters. There's a huge range in traditional Italian dishes, ranging from light Mediterranean-style seafood dishes from the south with light tomato-based sauces to heavy, creamy pasta

---

≞🍴 Question: Why doesn't every restaurant provide nutrition information?

Answer: They claim it'd be difficult to do, but it wouldn't.

Actually, many restaurants want to encourage people to indulge because overstuffed customers are happy customers. Also, people generally hate thinking about the consequences of an indulgence while they're "treating" themselves, and restaurants will do anything they can to make people feel removed from that. This situation will all change someday soon, though.

The future of calorie counting is very bright. Within a decade, I expect the law will make it possible to get a close-to-accurate calorie count on almost everything sold at restaurants. It might even be printed on the menu!

New York City fired the first shots in this war in 2008 when the Board of Health voted to require restaurants with fifteen or more outlets to post calorie counts on their menus; sadly, that's only about 10 percent of all the city's restaurants.

That policy went federal in March 2010. As part of the sweeping health reform law colloquially known as Obama-

---

dishes. Let's look at Olive Garden for our calorie counts—not because it's good, but because it's easy to compare with what you'll find on the menu at most other Italian sit-down joints.

The first problem with Italian restaurants like Olive Garden is that the portions are usually huge. If you can muster the discipline to ask for a box when your entrée arrives, that's a great move, and I salute you. I find it easier just to order something I can finish without downing too many calories. The second problem is all the free and warm bread—you've

---

care, every restaurant chain with more than twenty locations will be forced to post calorie information on their menus and drive-through signs. The law should be in effect in 2011.

Almost all of the nutrition information that will be revealed by the law is already available, of course. Either because the restaurant released it or a publication like *Nutrition Action* has retrieved it by other some means. So this really isn't a huge deal for you and me. We want every restaurant to do it because we're aware ignorance is not bliss.

So why should the disclosure laws stop with chain restaurants? Chances are, the big chains' powerful congressional lobby won't let the laws hurt their business without other restaurants bearing the brunt, which means sometime down the road we can expect similar measures affecting all restaurants, big and small. Despite claims to the contrary, they have a pretty good idea what they're putting in their dishes. Restaurants strive for consistency, so it's not as if they're deliberately allowing a big variance in the plates they're sending out of the kitchen. Also, many of the ingredients they buy already come in labeled packages for *their* convenience. Really, there's no good excuse.

gotta set that basket aside, since a single slice can be about 100 calories without butter or olive oil.

The Best and Most Responsible Choice: Every Italian restaurant I've ever visited has salads, so be sure to start with one of those topped with the lightest dressing they have. Olive Garden's salad is known to be pretty good, and it's fairly light either with dressing (360 calories) or without (120 calories). Grilled chicken and fish dishes are often the safest way to go when they're available. Olive Garden's Parmesan-Crusted Tilapia (590 calories) demonstrates why. Good old-fashioned spaghetti with meat sauce (710 calories) is also a decent choice so long as you avoid the version with meatballs (1,110 calories) or, worse yet, sausage (1,270 calories).

A Minor Indulgence: Lasagna is filled with cheese and sometimes covered in meat, but at 850 calories it's not too terrible, especially if you can eat half with a salad and take the other half home. Chicken Marsala (770 calories) also isn't too bad. Remember that anything fried or cheesy—that means entrées called "Parmigiana" or "Alfredo"—can be heavier than you'd expect. Eggplant Parmesan sounds pretty innocuous (it's just eggplant!), but at 850 calories it's not as light as it may seem.

Dear God, No: Though it's technically seafood, fried calamari (1,070 calories) is no calorie bargain thanks to the breading and oil. Fettuccine Alfredo (1,220 calories) is the poster child for "Bad Italian Pick," thanks to the thick noodles and rich cheese.

MIDDLE EASTERN/GREEK

Keep in Mind: You know all that stuff about the "good fats" in olives and feta cheese? Forget about it for now. When you're losing weight, there's no such thing as "healthy but high-calorie foods," which means you need to be very careful what you eat in the realm of Middle Eastern and Greek cuisine. There are a number of tasty options, but you're going to have to limit some of the best parts.

Nutrition information for this section comes from Pita Jungle, an Arizona chain that's not only incredibly delicious but also pretty similar to what you'll find at most sit-down Med restaurants. Props to them for posting nutrition information, which isn't always pretty given their huge portions. Still, Pita Jungle's portions are pretty well in line with what I see people eating at similar restaurants, so it's good of them to come forward with their numbers.

The Best and Most Responsible Choice: A chicken shawarma wrap (650 calories) is my default choice at any Middle Eastern restaurant, as it's a lot lighter than a beef or lamb gyro (800 calories). A small Greek salad (330 calories with dressing) is nice on the side. If you see a tasty salad with grilled or broiled chicken, get that with the dressing on the side, and you could save several hundred calories.

A Minor Indulgence: For me, it's the appetizers. There are about 25 calories per tablespoon in hummus (tabouli and baba ghanoush are fairly similar), so be sure to split the order with someone and try to use only half a pita (there are 250 calories in a large pita).

Dear God, No: Steer clear of the deep-fried falafel (500 calories), the bread, the olive oil, and the cheese. Also be aware that olive oil has a massive 120 calories per tablespoon, so actively avoid consuming any more than you have to.

EASTERN EUROPEAN

Keep in Mind: As you can probably tell from my surname (it means "shoemaker" in Slovak), I have central and eastern European roots. There aren't a lot of restaurants that brand themselves as Russian or Czech or Polish, sadly, but I wanted to include this section to clear up common misconceptions about the healthfulness of the diet in nations formerly part of, or bordering, the USSR.

The Best and Most Responsible Choice: Goulash, a type of soup popular in Hungary, Slovakia, and other Slavic nations, is similar in calories to beef stew or chili. The main ingredients are meat, onions, paprika, and sometimes potatoes, which means that the only calorie-killer could be fatty meat. Ask how lean their meat is, but count on about 300 calories for a large cup. Sometimes it's served with pasta, which could quickly double that calorie count.

A Minor Indulgence: Pierogies, half moon–shaped dumplings filled with mashed potatoes that are found across central and eastern Europe, are not bad so long as they're boiled or baked instead of fried and not covered with butter or sour cream. For reference, the supermarket variety with cheese, from Mrs. T's, has 60 calories each. If you order them in a restaurant, ask if they're boiled and scrape off any creamy toppings.

Dear God, No: Any sort of sausage is a bad, bad choice. There's no such thing as a lean or low-cal sausage, especially not at a restaurant.

MEXICAN

Keep in Mind: Mexican food is often unjustly maligned for perceived unhealthiness, but it isn't so. Sure, you can binge on refried beans and rice covered in cheese and walk out of the neighborhood cantina having consumed a full day's calories, but it's also easy to find light and fresh items on the menu at most sit-down Mexican joints.

For this one I'm pulling nutrition information from Chevys Fresh Mex, a California chain with a decent reputation. Now, it's probably worth noting that I've never been to Chevys, even though there is one less than a mile from my home. Sorry, but in Arizona it's sort of a crime to not go local when you're eating Mexican. Still, from what I hear, it's about what you'll get most places.

The Best and Most Responsible Choice: Tacos are almost always the way to go with Mexican food. They're simple, flavorful, and you can see everything that's in them and peel off what you don't want (read: slice of avocado, 50 calories). Street taco style—just meat, onions, cilantro, and a squeeze of lime on a corn tortilla—is the way to go if you can get them, but a sprinkling of cheese won't kill you. Chicken (280 calories) is lighter than carnitas (360 calories) or beef (290 calories), but go with what you like and limit yourself to one or two. A side of black beans (190 calories) or Mexican rice (180 calories) is a lot better than refried beans (280 calories).

A Minor Indulgence: Fajitas aren't really anything like actual Mexican food, but if you've got a craving (I often do), know that a plate of either steak or chicken fajitas and vegetables sautéed in oil comes in at around 1,000 calories. Also worth noting, most restaurants' tortilla chips are about 20 calories each, so go easy on them and dip each one deeply into the salsa—you can consume a pound of salsa for less than 100 calories.

Dear God, No: Quesadillas are the ultimate diet-killer. Since they're essentially just cheese and meat stuffed inside a tortilla and pan-fried, they're not the most filling option, and you're looking at a minimum of 1,200 calories. If you add guacamole (about 130 calories per ounce) or sour cream (60 calories per ounce), you're really sabotaging yourself. It should go without saying that enchiladas, which are covered in thick sauce and cheese, and chimichangas (deep-fried burritos) are poor choices.

ETHIOPIAN

Keep in Mind: Ethiopian food tends to be fairly light and filling—even though you use carb-heavy injera, a thin bread with a pancake-like consistency, to scoop up the entrées instead of silverware. Greens and cabbage are at the center of the menu and are very light so long as the restaurant doesn't flavor them with a lot of niter kebbeh, the spiced butter that is as essential to nearly every Ethiopian dish as berbere, their signature spice blend. Most Ethiopian foods are just different combinations of the house spice blends and either cabbage, collard greens, lentils, beef, chicken, potatoes, or lamb. That means you should order according to the main ingredient and hope for the best with the butter and spices.

For example, a cup of plain cooked lentils has about 220 calories. A cup of cooked cabbage, on the other hand, has only about 40 calories. Collard greens have 50 calories per cup. Boiled potatoes have about 140 calories per cup. Roasted chicken has about 230 calories per cup. Lamb is closer to 300 calories per cup. This information is what you need to decipher an Ethiopian menu.

Be on guard against overindulging, since the communal serving style typical of most Ethiopian restaurants offers the option of unintentionally bogarting the beg tibs.

The Best and Most Responsible Choice: About a half cup each of doro wat (spicy chicken, about 200 calories) and gomen wat (greens, about 100 calories) along with a few scoops of salad (80 calories if doused with oil) plus a 10-inch square of injera (400 calories). (That's an average I found from online recipes; obviously, each restaurant's injera varies.)

A Minor Indulgence: A half cup of the misir wat (lentils, about 250 calories) and tibs wot (potatoes, 270 calories) along with bread and salad.

Dear God, No: The lamb used at a lot of Ethiopian restaurants (anything with "beg" or "yebeg" in the name) tends to be pretty fatty and should be avoided as the lamb itself is probably around 300 calories per cup before butter and spices are added. Also refrain from going back for a second piece of injera—remember, that's probably an extra 400 calories.

CHINESE

Keep in Mind: When people say, "Asian food is healthy," they actually mean that Asian food *besides the stuff you typically find at most Chinese restaurants* is healthy. So much American Chinese food is fried, using cheap cuts of meat, with disastrous results. On the other hand, it is pretty ubiquitous, and there are even chains large enough to give us reliable nutrition information, which makes it a lot easier to figure out what you're getting. I'm pulling these numbers from a giant national chain, P.F. Chang's China Bistro, based in suburban Phoenix, where I live. The menu probably isn't much different from what you'll find around the corner from your place. A word of caution, however: Chang's breaks its menu down into multiple "servings" per dish, so the plate you get could have triple the calories of the first number you see. Pretty sneaky, I know, so watch out.

The Best and Most Responsible Choice: Moo Goo Gai Pan (610 calories), which you can find at most Chinese restaurants, is almost always a safe bet. Likewise, Ginger Chicken with Broccoli (620 calories) is a great pick.

A Minor Indulgence: Beef with Broccoli can be a smart pick from a Chinese restaurant, but Chang's (870 calories) shows it's not always super low-cal. Oddly, the Lo Mein Chicken (810 calories) is lighter but not as light as the Lo Mein Vegetable (560 calories). Don't count on this everywhere, though. Also, veggie dishes aren't light if they're made with coconut milk, as shown by the Coconut-Curry Vegetables (950 calories).

Dear God, No: Though chicken is very light, duck is very fatty and should almost always be avoided. Chang's Cantonese Roasted Duck (1,160 calories) shows why. Also avoid anything with the words "crispy," "orange," or something that sounds like a Bruce Lee movie: Chang's Crispy Honey Shrimp (860 calories), Orange Peel Chicken (1,090 calories), and Kung Pao Chicken (1,230). Try to skip appetizers in general, but whatever you do, don't ever order Chinese-style spare ribs (1,410 calories).

THAI

Keep in Mind: Thai food is very light so long as you avoid the heavy sauces and go easy on the rice and noodles. Try to find dishes that have as little sauce and as many vegetables as possible, and don't be shy about asking your waiter for light recommendations since a lot of dishes sound more innocuous than they actually are. Most Thai curries have coconut milk, a real calorie count killer at 80 calories per ounce, so steer clear of it unless you're budgeting for a higher-calorie meal. Thai peanut sauce is very high in calories, 35 per teaspoon, so pass on that, too.

The Best and Most Responsible Choice: Thai basil chicken can be found at almost any Thai restaurant and has tons of flavor from calorie-free spices for only about 250 calories per cup. Most of those calories actually come from the meat, with the number bumped up to account for oil, soy sauce (20 calories per ounce), and fish sauce (15 calories per ounce). Plan on adding 250 calories for a cup of steamed white rice.

A Minor Indulgence: A cup of a typical Thai chicken curry has about 340 calories. A 1-ounce stick of satay pork or a

1-ounce veggie spring roll is only about 100 calories, so if you're doing an appetizer, that's the way to go. Skip the dipping sauces. If you have a burning urge to dip your appetizers in something, try straight Sriracha, the hot sauce with a rooster on the bottle. Chances are, you can't consume more than 20 or 30 calories of that stuff without losing your appetite.

Dear God, No: A lot of massaman curries have both coconut milk *and* peanuts in them—you could be looking at 600-plus calories for a cup of one of those before you add rice.

VIETNAMESE

Keep in Mind: Vietnamese cuisine is extremely diverse, with age-old native dishes tweaked according to heavy Chinese and French influences. There are far too many signature dishes associated with Vietnamese cuisine to get into here, but we'll look at a few to seek and a few to avoid.

The Best and Most Responsible Choice: Pho, a traditional soup consisting of beef broth, thin slices of meat, and rice noodles served with an assortment of fresh herbs and sliced veggies like basil, bean sprouts, jalapeños, lime wedges, and cilantro, is always a nice treat. A nutritionist writing for *USA Today* reports that a large bowl of pho, which is incredibly filling, has 655 calories. I'm not sure how she got that number, but it seems pretty reasonable to me, so let's pin it on her. That's right: Get whatever meat you want—meatballs, brisket, chicken, or a combo thereof—and count it as 655 calories, courtesy of *USA Today*. Just kidding; stick with chicken or lean beef. Goi ga, a Vietnamese salad made with shredded cabbage, grilled chicken, and some herbs, is incredibly light except for the crushed peanuts and dressing—plan on about 450 calories if you go easy on the dressing.

A Minor Indulgence: If you're at a restaurant where they serve bánh mì, traditional Vietnamese sandwiches, know that they're actually lighter than pho. That makes them a great choice if you can find them and you don't get anything on the side. LA-based Lee's Sandwiches is the titan of the bánh mì world and publishes nutrition information, which earns them a plug here. Lee's grilled pork sandwich (300 calories) is amazingly decadent, considering it has fewer calories than many of Jared's favorite subs. The pate (430 calories) is a little more indulgent, but totally worth it. Vietnamese sandwiches have a lot in common with Subway, actually. They're baked on light and fluffy baguettes that appear to be a lot more substantial than they actually are, just like Subway's house-baked bread, and they tend to use lighter meats along with flavorful vegetables. When you get sick of the oven-roasted chicken breast sub, check them out.

Dear God, No: Chow fun, a wide rice noodle, isn't that awful in the grand scheme of things, but it's pretty bad compared to other Vietnamese food. A cup of cooked chow fun noodles is about 175 calories, which gets much worse if they're stir-fried or topped with pork—you could easily be looking at 800 calories for fried chow fun with a few pieces of meat.

JAPANESE

Keep in Mind: Traditional Japanese food tends to be very low in calories, even with the rice. Well, most of it, anyway. Sushi is great, of course, and Japanese-style steaks and chicken are also pretty light. The obvious exception is deep-fried tempura. Stick to sushi and lean meats along with small portions of rice.

Benihana is, as best I can tell, one of the few restaurants to actually have its nutrition information outed by New York City's new requirement. Most other chains didn't need Bloomberg and the boys to open them up, but Benihana did. You can't get calorie counts on the chain sushi and steak joint's main site, as best I can tell, unless you come in through a side door, specifically the New York City location's page. It's all laid out there, though, so we'll use them in honor of their reluctant support. Thanks, guys.

The Best and Most Responsible Choice: A California Roll (330 calories for the full) is always a safe bet, but a Tuna Roll (380 calories for the full) feels more substantial to me. If you'd prefer to dispense with the rice, you can pop pieces of tuna sashimi (20 calories), squid sashimi (10 calories), or salmon sashimi (35 calories) all night. Sushi and a side salad with tangy ginger dressing (90 calories) make for a nice meal. Add a cup of miso (40 calories)—which they oddly don't have at Benihana—for a nice light meal at your neighborhood sushi joint.

A Minor Indulgence: Japanese steakhouses are pretty easy on the calorie calculator, but don't go crazy with the meat—it adds up quickly. Hibachi chicken (280 calories) or steak (240 calories) aren't bad alone, but the combo plate puts you over 500 calories. Also plan on allotting about 560 calories for your share of rice and veggies from the grill.

Dear God, No: Beware of fried food and eel. The vegetable tempura appetizer (520 calories) is on a par with an entire steak and chicken meal. The Dragon Roll (570 calories), which has eel in it, isn't nearly as light as the tuna or crab rolls. In fact, a slice of eel sashimi (60 calories) is equal to three pieces of tuna.

INDIAN

Keep in Mind: Indian cuisine comes from the second most populous country on earth, a nation of 1.2 billion people speaking several hundred languages and cooking from millions of recipes. It's absolutely impossible to predict what you'll get in any local Indian restaurant because, while the names of dishes might be similarly Americanized, the actual ingredients can vary quite a bit.

In general, you're looking for baked entrées without heavy sauces, and you'll need to limit the amount of bread or rice you eat. Thankfully, a lot of Indian restaurants explain each menu item fairly extensively, so it's easy to avoid coconut milk–based curries and fried bread appetizers.

The Best and Most Responsible Choice: Chicken tikka is both ubiquitous and consistently low in calories. It's baked in a tandoor oven with spices and a butter glaze (called ghee) and topped with a thin yogurt sauce, leaving it succulent but relatively light. As a calorie reference, check out the frozen Chicken Tikka Masala from Trader Joe's (300 calories). Chances are, you'll get at least twice the amount of meat and rice at a restaurant, and there may well be more butter and yogurt in it, so budget at least 600 calories. Using the frozen food method is smart for anything not mentioned here, by the way. Large ethnic grocers sell frozen versions of pretty much any food you'll find in an ethnic restaurant, and it's easy to eyeball them and note what's in your favorite dishes for reference when ordering out.

A Minor Indulgence: I love naan bread, but given that a slice of naan has at least 200 calories (and up to 400), it's a lot smarter to plan on the basmati rice. Indian rice is closer to 200 calories for an entire cup—a very filling portion. For an entrée, tandoori chicken is always a nice choice; it's baked in a thin sauce, but the portions tend to be pretty large (recipes suggest 250 calories for a breast, 300 calories for a leg and thigh), and without any vegetables or sauce it's not as filling as the tikka.

Dear God, No: Avoid yogurt, all the glorious breads, and curries made with coconut. Any of the breads will be bad, but the malpua (800 calories), a sweet, fritter-style treat, may be the worst.

DINERS

Keep in Mind: There may not be anything that separates the young and hip from the old and lame more than Sunday brunch. I mean, really, what says "I'm young and cool and without serious obligations" more than sitting around and leisurely drinking cup after cup of coffee while dishing dirt about the previous night's festivities? So, yeah, eating a big diner breakfast is a big calorie commitment, but you may well need to make such a commitment from time to time to avoid alienating your friends.

You probably know a great little place you like to go, but for the sake of universality we'll look at calorie counts from Denny's. Perhaps more than anywhere else, what you tell the waitress at a diner makes all the difference. Short-order cooks are amazingly adaptable and can make two dishes that have the same name and the same price but differ exponentially in calories. Beware that most diners use three or four eggs per omelet, fry that omelet in oil, and top it with a half cup of cheese or more, putting them around 1,000 calories instead of the 400 or so you'd get from egg whites and veggies without the cheese.

Remember that orange juice (122 calories per 8-ounce glass) is nominally "healthy" but not diet-friendly. Go with coffee or tea and artificial sweetener; one little brown packet of Sugar in the Raw, which any hipster diner will have, is 20 calories. If you want creamer, count 20 calories for each little peel-top cup. That really adds up as "Barb" or "Alice" pours you three or four cups during the two hours you take up space in the booth she desperately wants to turn over for a second tip. (An aside: At diners, it's kosher to double your tip for every half hour you stay after the first hour. That's the Chubster way.)

Be careful about breakfast cocktails. Add a little champagne to your orange juice and you're starting the day pretty far behind—150 calories for one small mimosa. If you've gotta have the hair of the dog, a Bloody Mary is made with tomato juice, which is much, much lighter than orange juice (50 calories for 8 ounces), and vodka. It packs much more of a punch for 122 calories.

But skip the cocktails if you can and try to order things that are light on cheese and meat and come in sensible, easily identifiable portions.

The Best and Most Responsible Choice: Build Your Own Grand Slam with oatmeal (280 calories), turkey bacon (70 calories), seasonal fruit (70 calories), and two scrambled egg whites (50 calories).

A Minor Indulgence: A veggie cheese omelet (460 calories) with hash browns (210 calories) and grits (220 calories).

Dear God, No: Bananas Foster French Toast Skillet (860 calories) with sausage links (370 calories).

Stuff You Can Barely Afford: Upscale Restaurants

Generally speaking, fine dining establishments are a waste of time and money for dieters—especially if they're French. While it may be true that French women don't get fat, Americans who eat too many baguettes and lots of foie gras do. People go to restaurants like this because they want to splurge, both financially and calorically, and that isn't the mind frame you should be in right now. The experience of eating at almost any restaurant aspiring to earn a Michelin star is wrapped up in the decadence of the food, which is the exact sort of situation you want to avoid. How many "foodies" do you know who are plumping up a bit? Probably a few. If, however, you end up in one of these places, there are some things you can order besides whatever newfangled version of a salad, baked potato, and lean steak they're peddling.

The downside of dining at upscale eateries is that they do pretty much everything they can to distinguish themselves from other places, rather than just making the best version of conventional dishes they know you and I will order, as is customary in casual sit-down joints. This makes it hard to know what to order since there are all sorts of traps—you could easily order a dish that sounds as if it should be mostly made of spinach and end up with a creamy sauce on top.

The upshot is that they use a lot of the same ingredients—foodstuffs deemed either fancy or trendy enough for the palates of the well-heeled customers who keep these joints in business by eating there consistently while you and I just drop by for birthday dinners and other special occasions. Once you decode the list of exotic ingredients, finding a low-cal meal to order becomes pretty simple.

So let's look at the ingredients you'll find in restaurants with trained chefs in white outfits. For the record, pretty much every word here was pulled off the menu of someplace that won a James Beard Award in 2009 and 2010, including places like the French Laundry, Craft, and the Slanted Door. If you've never looked through the menus at ten or twenty high-end restaurants, you should—it's amazing how much the ingredients overlap. Everyone loves a trend, it seems.

Here are some words you'll encounter and items to seek or avoid:

Aioli: Just a combination of olive oil, eggs, and garlic. That means it's always very high in calories. Avoid.

Arugula: This leaf vegetable is used in many salads because it has a lot more flavor than other salad greens. There are fewer than 10 calories in a cup of the stuff. Seek.

Barramundi: An Australian/Asian fish popular in Thai fusion foods. It's a white, flaky fish often steamed or baked and flavored with herbs like lemongrass and garlic. A large fillet will likely be only about 200 calories. Seek.

Braised: Think of braising as a French version of Dutch oven cooking. The food is seared, then slow-cooked in juice. What you get out of it depends on what you put in the pot, so look for braised vegetables and leaner types of meat. Seek.

Brussels sprouts: A common type of cabbage you may remember avoiding as a child. They're very rich in nutrients and only about 15 calories per ounce. However, they can also be topped with a lot of butter, which is something to ask your waiter about. Seek with caution.

Bucatini: Just hollow spaghetti noodles. Avoid.

Capers: The pickled buds of the caper bush are used in a lot of Southern Italian cuisine. They pack a ton of flavor into very few calories, less than 10 per ounce. Seek.

Capicola: Fancy bacon. Avoid.

Caviar: These sturgeon roe (aka fish eggs) are synonymous with the lifestyles of the rich and famous. Caviar is about 70 calories per ounce, but feel free to eat what you can afford. Seek.

Chorizo: This extremely fatty Spanish sausage has made its way from tapas bars into all sorts of fusion food. It's intensely flavorful in small amounts and can be OK in that context, but don't order anything that uses it as the main protein. Avoid.

Crème fraîche: This fancy sour cream is made with milk high in butterfat. Eat it just as often as you would regular American sour cream, which is almost never. Avoid.

Crostini: These are just little pieces of toast. They're the caloric equivalent of giant croutons and are often drizzled with oil or butter. Avoid.

Duck: Duck is a fatty, calorie-heavy dish. Avoid.

Emulsion: Culinary emulsions usually involve oil or egg yolks. Avoid.

Endive: A delicious leaf vegetable that's very low in calories. Seek.

Fennel: A Mediterranean vegetable, it's a flavorful addition to a lot of healthy dishes. Seek.

Foie gras: Fatted duck or goose liver. It has more than 100 calories per ounce. Avoid.

Frisée: See endive.

Gnocchi: Dumpling-like pasta often made with potato. It is delicious but has more than 250 calories per cup. Avoid.

Halibut: A lean but very flavorful fish. Count around 400 calories for a large fillet. Seek.

Idiazabal: A Spanish cheese made from unpasteurized sheep's milk. Avoid.

Jamón serrano: Fancy bacon. Avoid.

Jidori chicken: A special kind of Japanese organic free-range chicken. Count it the same as normal chicken. Seek.

Kale: A mineral-rich kind of cabbage that is supertrendy with food bloggers right now. Seek.

Leeks: A fancy cousin to onions and garlic, they are very flavorful with few calories unless sautéed in oil. Seek.

Lychee: This Chinese fruit is low in calories. Seek.

Mascarpone: A spreadable, soft Italian cheese. Avoid.

Mizuna: A Japanese green similar to arugula. Seek.

Molasses: A byproduct of processed sugar. Very high in calories. Avoid.

Mousse: A mousse is a kind of foam popular in French cuisine. Not all mousses are sweet desserts full of sugar or chocolate, but most use heavy cream to attain the desired consistency. Even a savory spinach mousse should probably be avoided, as it was likely made with thick, high-calorie cream. Avoid.

New potatoes: The same as old potatoes in terms of calories. Seek.

Oxtail: A cut of beef that is usually slow-cooked and often incorporated into a soup. At less than 50 calories per ounce, it's comparable to a lot of lean beef. Seek.

Oysters: Very low in calories if broiled (10 each) and very high in calories (50 each) if fried. Seek and avoid accordingly.

Pancetta: Fancy bacon. Avoid.

Pecorino: A hard Italian cheese made with sheep's milk. Hard cheeses are lower in fat than softer, richer cheeses, and their intense flavor lends itself to smaller portion sizes. Seek with caution.

Persimmon: One of several varieties of fruit found in American, Asian, and Mediterranean cuisine. It's often used in desserts and puddings that are high in calories and should be avoided, but it can also occasionally be found fresh or dried in salads. Seek.

Polenta: This Italian dish made of boiled cornmeal is very high in calories. Expect up to 500 per cup. Considering that it's often served with sausage, this is one to pass on. Avoid.

Pomegranate: This fruit is naturally very low in calories, but, in culinary use, it is usually reduced and sweetened into a Kool-Aid-like paste. Avoid.

Porchetta: A very fatty type of Italian roasted pork. Avoid.

Prosciutto: Fancy bacon. Avoid.

Quinoa: A South American grain that is very nutritious but, at close to 100 calories per ounce, not a great diet food. Avoid.

Ragù: Note the accent, which is how you know it's not the brand of spaghetti sauce sold at most American supermarkets. Ragù is actually the Italian word for a meat-based sauce—not necessarily very high in calories if the meat is lean but probably more than a simple, fresh tomato, basil, and garlic sauce. Avoid.

Rapini: A cousin of broccoli often used in Italian food. Seek.

Risotto: This is an Italian rice dish that is very creamy, partly because of the cooking method and partly because cheese is usually added. Expect about 350 calories per serving. Avoid.

Scallions: These mild green onions are very low in calories unless sautéed in olive oil. Seek with caution.

Shallots: Fancy onions. Seek.

Sorbet: This sweetened and frozen fruit juice is a lot lighter than ice cream (the Häagen-Dazs version has 220 calories per cup—less than half of what their ice cream promises) but not something to go crazy with. Seek.

Sweetbreads: These are either the neck or pancreas of some animal that's been poached in milk, then breaded and fried. I don't eat them; you shouldn't, either. Avoid.

Truffles: Extremely expensive mushrooms. Pretty innocuous, diet-wise. Truffle oil, the cheaper substitute, on the other hand, is made mainly with olive oil and is high in calories. Seek or avoid accordingly.

Unagi: Japanese freshwater eel, often served in sushi rolls or as sashimi, which is much fattier than fish. Avoid.

Veal: The meat of a young calf is sort of out of vogue right now but could come back at any time. If roasted or grilled, its 50 calories per ounce is not much more than regular beef, though much more tender. Seek.

Vinaigrette: This mixture of vinegar and oil is usually used for salads. It varies widely in calorie content depending on the proportion of vinegar (10 calories per tablespoon for Balsamic) to oil (120 calories per tablespoon for olive). Don't order it unless it's presented as the "light" option. Avoid.

Watercress: This leaf vegetable has very few calories. Seek.

XO Sauce: A thick and spicy Chinese fish sauce that has 80 calories per tablespoon. Avoid.

Xocolatl: The Aztec word for chocolate. Just as many calories as regular chocolate. Avoid.

Yellowfin: A species of tuna, also known as ahi. Wonderful seared or raw. About 40 calories per ounce. Seek.

Zabaione: This Italian dessert custard is made with egg yolks, sugar, and sweet wine. Very high in calories. Avoid.

Stuff You Can Cook (That's Super Fast and Easy)

I am not much of a cook. *At all.* Whatever culinary aspirations I once had—mainly manifested in a long-running dinner club I formed with two neighbors in Virginia that saw me cooking such delicacies as bacon-topped, blue cheese–stuffed burgers and 2,500-calorie taco salads—seem to have died when my weight-loss project started.

There are so many other things I'd rather do than cook, especially given that I'm not very good at it. Also, my girlfriend, Kirsten, is a great cook with her own little food blog

(MyFirstThyme.blogspot.com) and takes on projects like reverse-engineering the best salsa we've ever had by isolating the spices in it. I'm fortunate enough to benefit from her talents while limiting my own contributions to what can be done with a sponge and a dishtowel.

A million sources offer great recipes for dieters—*Cooking Light* magazine and the low-cal sections of allrecipes.com and eatingwell.com have been good to us—and I can't compete with them. So I won't try here.

However, in case you want to get your feet wet with low-cal cooking, here are five quick recipes to start you off. They are ranked by ascending difficulty, but they're all very easy and very cheap to make. Give them a try when you get bored with microwave meals and takeout joints.

SUPER-LIGHT TACO SALAD

I invented this myself. There are only about 100 calories in this entire meal.

2 cups Fresh Express Field Greens salad mix or similar
¼ cup fresh salsa from the refrigerated case at the
    supermarket
1 cheese-flavored rice cake, smashed into 1-inch bits

Put the salad greens on a plate and toss with the salsa. Top with the crumbled rice cakes for crunch and a hint of cheesiness.

FOUR-BEAN SALAD

This is my healthier variation of one of my mom's recipes—a very well balanced blend of protein and fiber. The entire

mix has about 650 calories, depending on the brand of salad
dressing you use, but you can get two meals out of it.

    1 can cut green beans
    1 can cut wax beans
    ½ can chickpeas
    ½ can kidney beans
    ¼ cup finely chopped onion
    ½ cup finely chopped green pepper
    ½ cup low-calorie Italian dressing
    ¼ cup apple cider vinegar
    5 packets artificial sweetener
    Hot sauce to taste (I prefer about 3 tablespoons
        Sriracha)

Drain the canned beans and mix together in a storage container. Stir in the onion and green pepper. Mix the Italian dressing and vinegar together and stir in the sweetener
until it dissolves. Combine the dressing with the bean mixture, shake well, and refrigerate for at least 2 hours before
serving.

BAKED KALE CHIPS

This is Kirsten's adaptation of a recipe that's all over the
Internet. The only real calories here are from the olive oil,
which has about 120 calories.

    1 bunch kale
    1 tablespoon olive oil
    1 teaspoon salt

1. Preheat the oven to 350 degrees. Line a cookie sheet with
parchment paper.

2. Remove the thick stems from the kale and tear into bite-sized pieces. Wash and dry thoroughly. In a bowl, toss the kale together with the olive oil and salt.

3. Spread in a single layer on the cookie sheet and bake until the edges are brown but not burned, 10–15 minutes.

POOR MAN'S GOI GA

This is my cheap knockoff of a favorite salad from a Vietnamese restaurant in Scottsdale, Arizona. The dressing is light and tasty and matches the restaurant version very well. The noodles are the only higher-calorie component, but a half block is only about 190 calories. The 250-calorie chicken breast and 120 calories of dressing put the total with vegetables at less than 600 calories, making this a very filling and well-balanced meal.

1 boneless, skinless chicken breast, cut into slices
½ block chicken-flavor ramen noodles
¼ cup Kraft Light Asian Toasted Sesame dressing
½ head Napa cabbage
1 carrot
¼ bunch cilantro

1. Cook the chicken and ramen noodles using your preferred method. Use the entire seasoning packet, but toss out half the noodles—even if you're wasting a dime's worth of food. Shred the chicken, combine with the noodles and salad dressing, and refrigerate for a few hours if possible.

2. Shred the cabbage and carrot and finely chop the cilantro. Put the vegetables on a large plate. Place the chilled chicken, noodles, and dressing over the vegetables and serve.

ROASTED CAULIFLOWER AND RED PEPPER SOUP

This is Kirsten's adaptation of a recipe from Closet Cooking (www.closetcooking.com). Depending on the kind of stock you use and how much yogurt you add, plan on about 250 calories per cup. Makes 2 servings.

1 head cauliflower, cut into florets
2 large red bell peppers, roughly chopped
3 tablespoons olive oil
Salt and pepper
1 white onion, chopped
2 cloves garlic, minced
½ teaspoon cayenne pepper
3 cups chicken or vegetable stock
½ cup plain Greek yogurt

1. Preheat the oven to 400 degrees.
2. Toss the cauliflower and bell pepper pieces in 2 tablespoons of the olive oil. Season with salt and pepper to taste and arrange in a single layer in a flameproof baking dish. Roast until the cauliflower is lightly golden brown, 20–30 minutes.
3. Heat the remaining tablespoon of olive oil in a pan. Add the onion and sauté until tender, 5–7 minutes. Add the garlic and sauté for about 30 seconds.
4. Transfer the onion and garlic to the baking dish and add the cayenne and stock. Bring to a boil, reduce the heat, cover, and simmer until the cauliflower is tender, about 20 minutes.
5. Puree with a hand blender or food processor. Serve, garnished with a dollop of Greek yogurt in the center of each bowl.

ALCOHOL AND DRUGS

Abstainer: A weak person who yields to the temptation of denying himself a pleasure. —AMBROSE BIERCE

FIRST, THE BAD NEWS: CALORIES MATTER EVEN WHEN THEY'RE in liquid form. You can sip, shake, stir, or funnel them, but if they find their way down your gullet, they still count. This applies to soda, milk shakes, and smoothies. More pressingly, it applies to booze. If you're dieting, you need to scrawl any calorie you drink—even a shot of whiskey or a warm half cup of light beer—in the tally right below wholesome consumables like oatmeal and apples. No excuses, no rationalizations, no forgetting.

That's not a reason to mope, though. You wanna party with some friends this weekend? You can totally do it, but you're going to have to budget accordingly.

Let's say it's Saturday morning and you're planning to hit a few bars and see a show later. This is the time to use the little tricks you've already learned for shaving calories, planning your day so you've got some wiggle room at sundown. Make a few key cuts, and you can easily have four or five drinks over the course of an evening. Provided they're the right sorts of drinks, of course. Still, not bad, right?

Oh, and let's not forget that your daily calorie count resets at midnight. That's a nice little loophole. So, if you're out late and the clock strikes twelve, you can eat (pun intended) into the new day's allotment with another drink or two—just plan on limiting yourself to a salad while watching *The Simpsons* on Sunday night.

But to make this work, you're going to need some willpower. It can be hard to make smart decisions when you're under the influence, but you need to if you want to make this diet work. Those smart decisions start with the commitment to not get too far under the influence, lest you be more easily overwhelmed by temptation. Can you handle it? I totally believe in you. But if you fuck up and eat a Sbarro slice around 2 A.M., you're going to need to reevaluate things. Maybe you need to lay off the sauce for a few months. That would suck, but if you can't handle your alcohol, you're gonna have to bite the bullet. Let's not have that happen.

The good news is that there are a lot of classic and totally reasonable drinks that don't have too many calories. Do you already like the stuff your grandpappy drank? You're in luck, as those tend to be the most diet-friendly drinks behind the bar. The bad news is that most of the girlie stuff—piña coladas, Mike's Hard Lemonade, Zima—is pretty much off the table. Do you drink a lot of that stuff now? Hopefully not. If so, this little diet plan is going to double as an occasion to refine and mature your palate so you can drink like a grownup. That's probably for the best anyway.

A Few Words on Boozing

The standard dieting advice about alcohol is pretty simple: Don't drink it. Seriously, it's amazing how often that little chestnut appears in ostensibly reputable sources of weight-loss advice, and it's even more surprising how many people seem satisfied with that answer. Actually, it's not so much "amazing" or "surprising" as it is "totally crazy." Just say no? Really? That's the best they've got?

Successful dieting, as we've discussed, is not about giving up any one thing that's supposedly responsible for your condition. There are no scapegoats; you just need to steadily undo your excesses. But in the meantime you still need to live your life, and for most of us that means tipping a few back from time to time.

True, not everyone in America drinks. Mormons, Muslims, and straight-edgers all refrain. As it happens, plenty of other people do, too. The proportion of Americans who drink has hovered around two thirds since pollsters started inquiring about it just before the start of World War II, which means that one third of the American populace does not drink—or at least won't admit they drink to a stranger on the telephone. Amazing, right? And you thought it was just uptight weirdoes, religious nuts, and Ian MacKaye!

Actually, nondrinkers are a little ahead of the game when it comes to the weight-loss thing. Not only does alcohol tend to have a lot of calories, it also tends to lower your inhibitions and make sticking to important life plans (read: your mission to stop being fat) harder. A number of unscientific but reproducible studies conducted last weekend at our nation's most respected universities confirm that alcohol makes many people very hungry for greasy, fried, cheesy, and sugary foods late at night. That's all bad, of course.

What I'm trying to say is that if you're harboring any puritanical or prohibitionist sympathies or have any interest in converting to a religion that will send you to hell for drinking, now is a great time to take the plunge and convert. Look for one of those awesome Christian fundamentalist sects where they don't take the Bible so literally as to serve actual wine at communion rather than grape juice but somehow still take it literally enough to believe the world was created in a mere seven days. If you choose this path, go ahead and skip to the next chapter! We'll see you again in a few pages, buddy.

A Few More Words on Boozing

And now, for the rest of us, some facts about how you can successfully drink and diet. First, let's look at what's at stake here.

There are very few politically relevant things in this book—that's an odd commonality in diet books—but the booze issue is one of them. I don't really want to go all culture warrior on you here, but in a time when certain other mind-altering substances are still illegal without any justification whatsoever, I feel compelled to point out that you have a constitutional right to drink. I mean, think about that: *They had to amend the United States Constitution to let you drink a beer.* That's pretty profound, right? So, yeah, not only *can* you drink while dieting; you *should* drink while dieting. The rest of us are counting on you to help preserve and protect the basic freedoms our forefathers won for us. Use them or lose them.

Furthermore, drinking while dieting is a good way to demonstrate to people, including yourself, that you're still living a normal life. You're not going to become an antisocial loser too obsessed with health to have a good time on this diet. You're just gracefully improving your health and appearance, not joining the circus. Friends don't need to pity or avoid you because you're making some lifestyle changes. Repeat after me: *It's not that big a deal, dude.*

So here's how to do it without sabotaging your weight-loss plans.

Light Beer: Not the Answer

It may come as a surprise to you if you're a big television watcher, with all the advertisements for ever-fancier super "light" beers and whatnot, but special diet beers are not the only solution to the drinking-while-dieting problem. They're sort of the worst, actually.

Let me note that this advice is given with the assumption that you want to get a little buzzed. Some people claim they drink for other reasons, but that's sort of weird and nonsensical to me. Why drink alcohol if you don't want to drink it in such a way that you feel the warm and fuzzy effect it often triggers, a phenomenon usually regarded as essential to the experience? So, yeah, let's definitely assume you want to feel your booze here—let's even go so far as to say that's the point of drinking—in which case the low-cal suds they're now selling are not necessarily gonna help you out.

I'll explain, using examples from the line of fine products sold by the hard-working people at Budweiser, makers of some of our nation's best-selling beers and sakes. (Budweiser "beer" is made with 30 percent rice—that makes it sake in my world.)

As you may know, Budweiser recently introduced a 55-calorie version of its Select beer. Dieters rejoiced—until they realized that 55-calorie beer is a mere 2.4 percent alcohol by volume. Regular Bud, by comparison, is 5 percent alcohol, which is pretty standard for mass-market American beer. At 2.4 percent, Bud Select 55 is actually more like the so-called low-point beer that some conservative states like Utah and Oklahoma make grocery stores sell instead of real beer or Budweiser-brand sake.

Let's leave taste aside for a moment and consider—on a purely calorie-oriented level—Bud Select 55, which has exactly half the calories of 110-calorie Bud Light. Bud Light is 4.2 percent alcohol. So, yes, Bud Select 55 is a *slightly* better deal. But not by any appreciable margin.

There are about 145 calories in a regular bottle of Budweiser, by the way, and it has 5 percent alcohol. So take a moment to consider whether light beer, stripped of all the marketing hokum, is really light? Is it really anything more than regular beer with more water in it, as the wise old men in your life have always alleged?

Sorta. Comparing calories to alcohol, Bud Light is about 10 percent "lighter" than Bud. Bud Select 55 is 12 percent lighter than Bud Light and 22 percent lighter than regular Budweiser.

Now let's go back and factor in taste and cost. After all, they're not charging half as much for a bottle of the 55-calorie stuff. You still want that super-light beer, fella?

Maybe we should consider outward appearances, too. Bud Light is socially acceptable in most circles, I guess, especially for the ladies. But what about Bud Select 55? True, I'm an insufferable beer snob (more on that later), but I probably wouldn't be the only one looking down on you for drinking that crap. Just keepin' it real, folks.

So, you might be wondering, does it even matter which Budweiser product I drink? Why should I even care?

The point here is certainly not to encourage fatalistic complacency—or, worse yet, drive you to the "no drinking on a diet" camp—but to get you to look at other options.

That is to say, consider Bud Ice.

It's sort of counterintuitive, given its slight sweetness, but Bud Ice—the much-maligned bargain brew—is actually the lightest beer Budweiser makes. That's right, Bud Ice isn't just for homeless alkies anymore, it's also Chubster approved! At 123 calories per serving and 5.5 percent alcohol, it's even better for a dieter looking for a buzz than Bud Select 55.

True, bottles of Bud Ice are probably not available at most bars, especially vaguely trendy ones, and I'm not sure they

---

🍺🍷🍸 Domestic Beers

SMART

Miller Lite	96 calories	4.2% alcohol
Natural Light	94 calories	4.2% alcohol
Rolling Rock	120 calories	4.5% alcohol

STUPID

Sam Adams Boston Lager	170 calories	4.9% alcohol
Old Milwaukee	146 calories	4.5% alcohol
Pabst Blue Ribbon	153 calories	5% alcohol

even sell it in kegs, but if you can find it, it's your best bet. Also, from an image standpoint, it's absolutely the coolest Budweiser there is. Bud Ice is sort of ironic, but not in the awful "Pimps and Hoes Frat Party" manner of most young white people drinking malt liquor. Bring your own bottle of Bud Ice to the next party you're hitting up. You will get drunk, and everyone will think you're cool and unique. That's the best you can hope for here, folks.

Budweiser-wise, at least.

Fancy Beer

Traditional wisdom holds that paler, lighter-bodied beers are better for dieters. "The darker the brew, the higher the calorie count" is an old axiom you've probably heard a few times. As it happens, that's not so much an extreme oversimplification as it is complete and total bullshit.

Actually, the opposite is often true. To make this point, let's look at a few run-of-the-mill imports you've probably drunk more than a few times.

First, consider Guinness Draught. Pretty dark, right? It's not quite coal-colored, but it's the darkest beer the average American ever drinks—and that's usually only once a year, while wearing a green T-shirt with lewd puns printed on it. But there are only about 125 calories in a 12-ounce bottle of the super-dark stout, which is 4.27 percent alcohol.

Now take Stella Artois. The name, translated from the Latin, means "star," and it sure is bright and sparkly. There are 150 calories in a bottle of the famous Belgian pilsner despite its light straw color. Sure, it has a little more alcohol by volume—5.2 percent—but the buzz-to-calorie ratio is still below what you'll get from a Guinness.

So, yes, Guinness is a much better dieting beer than Stella—and not because of any of those dubious health claims the Irish like to make about their minerals and vitamins and spring water and stuff.

The point is this: When counting your calories, you need to actually look at how each individual beer stacks up rather than resorting to frat house proverbs.

In terms of calories, beers vary hugely by style. The more sugar used to brew the style, the more calories the finished product will have. The calories in beer come mostly from either the actual alcohol or the sugars the yeast didn't gobble up and change into alcohol. When brewers make high-octane beers, they start with more sugar, some of which is converted to alcohol, and the rest of which remains in the bottle as sweetener. That's why a lot of superstrong beers—imperial IPAs, for example—are nearly as sweet as white wine despite the hefty dose of bittering hops added by brewers. All those sugars really pump up calorie counts, too. Take, for example, Dogfish Head's almost magical 120 Minute IPA, which is a staggering 18 percent alcohol and has an even more staggering 450 calories per 12-ounce serving. Eek. You should probably stick with the Dogfish Head 60 Minute IPA, which has fewer than half as many calories (209 per bottle) or with the brewery's surprisingly light Festina Peche, a beer brewed in a German style and made with real peaches that still manages to come in at 160 calories and about 4.5 percent alcohol.

As you can see, craft beer can be pretty complex on the calorie front. Something made with fresh fruit can be a decent choice, while a superstrong IPA will probably be a killer by any measure. If you're a beer snob—maybe, like me, you have a subscription to *BeerAdvocate*—you'll probably want to investigate this a bit on your own. In the meantime, remember that the sweeter the beer, the more calories it probably contains. Again, probably but not definitely. And style is only part of the equation.

Example: Sweet, fruity Blue Moon has 171 calories per bottle, meaning, by my rough estimate, that I probably had to lose about 10 pounds of pure Belgian-style *wit bier* during my diet. The very similar Goose Island 312 Urban Wheat, in contrast, has only 135 calories. Blue Moon is slightly more alcoholic, sure, but not nearly enough to justify those extra calories.

This can be a lot to keep track of, I know, but with many premium craft brews going for $15 a bottle and up, it's not a bad idea to take your time, do your research, and make smart picks.

Do you have a buddy who is brewing beer in his basement? So long as you trust his skills with the mash tun, there's no reason you need to abstain. Actually, any home brewer you

---

♟☕♟ Fancy Beers

SMART

Beck's Oktoberfest	135 calories	5.2% alcohol
Sapporo Premium	140 calories	4.9% alcohol
Deschutes Cascade Ale	140 calories	4.5% alcohol

STUPID

Anchor Porter	220 calories	5.6% alcohol
Leinenkugel's Berry Weiss	207 calories	4.7% alcohol
Pilsner Urquell	156 calories	4.4% alcohol

can trust to not make something that'll blind you will also be knowledgeable enough to tell you exactly how many calories are in his suds based on the gravity before and after fermentation. Homebrew geeks know these numbers, trust me.

It's a little too complicated for me to explain all the ins and outs here, but this is the equation to give him, courtesy of the American Society of Brewing Chemists:

The calories in a 12-ounce beer = [(6.9 x ABW) + 4.0 x (RE - 0.1)] x FG x 3.55.

The first item in brackets is the caloric contribution of the ethanol, which is determined from the alcohol by weight multiplied by 6.9 calories per gram of ethanol. The second bracket gives the caloric contribution of carbohydrates, which is determined by the Real Extract (calculated from the beginning and ending densities and 4 calories per gram for carbohydrates). The constant (0.1) accounts for the ash portion of the extract. The calories per 100 grams of beer is then converted to calories per 100 milliliters of beer by accounting for the final gravity and then to ounces.

Malt Liquor

Remember when I said that a higher alcohol content in beer usually means more calories per serving? That goes only for beers of the non–malt liquor variety. Malt liquor, as it turns out, could be the Chubster's best friend—if you pick one of the few really good choices.

Like regular beer, the stuff that comes in 40-ounce bottles is made primarily with barley, water, and hops. However, because it's aimed at budget-conscious consumers of mass qualities of alcohol (read: the homeless and otherwise downtrodden along with cheapskate college kids), makers of the type of beer commonly referred to as "malt liquor" also toss in cheap carbohydrates, like corn and rice. The idea is to get people fucked up as cheaply as legally possible. Their low-cal qualities are an ancillary benefit.

Consider this: Remember that old game Edward Forty-hands? You could play an entire game using King Cobra for about the same number of calories you'd find in a typical Chipotle burrito with meat, sour cream, and cheese. Seriously. King Cobra is 6 percent alcohol and has only 134 calories per 12-ounce serving. There are 6.6 servings in two 40-ounce bottles, which means that you could drink 80 ounces while consuming less than 900 calories. Am I saying you should do that? No, but if you do, please let me know how it turns out. Duct tape is optional.

Other malty brands in the 6 percent range, like Olde English 800 and Mickey's, are right around 160 calories per serving, so they're not always as good. The big boys, high-gravity 8 percent malts like Hurricane, St. Ides, and Steel Reserve, tend to be more than 200 calories per serving but are likely to make you sick before you can finish a bottle anyway.

♟☕♟ Malt Liquor

SMART

King Cobra	134 calories	6% alcohol
Hurricane High Gravity	186 calories	8.1% alcohol

STUPID

Mickey's	157 calories	5.6% alcohol
Milwaukee's Best Premium	128 calories	4.3% alcohol

Liquor

Now, if you're planning to cross that magical threshold from tipsy to drunk while holding fast to your calorie goal, you're probably going to need to do it with the help of liquor. There are a few exceptions, but the best calorie-to-alcohol ratios are generally found in the hard stuff.

The absolute best alcoholic beverage for dieters: Everclear. Although rarely consumed outside situations considered the traditional realm of roofies—that is to say, offered to under-age girls by creepy guys—Everclear is in a league of its own from a diet standpoint. In its purest form, it is 190 proof, which means that it's about 95 percent pure, unadulterated alcohol. Yes, there are 150 calories in a 1-ounce shot of the stuff. Here's the thing, though: That one shot has more al-cohol than two regular beers. So dilute your Everclear with diet soda, and you have a beverage that facilitates both drunkenness and weight loss.

Wanna hear something extra cool? Not only do diet soda mixers not have calories, they may actually help you get drunk faster than a regular soda! It's true. In 2006, Austra-lian researchers discovered that the compounds in common artificial sweeteners actually increase your body's rate of alcohol absorption, meaning that your body's peak blood-alcohol concentration will be "significantly higher" with a diet mixer than a regular one. In other words, a rum and diet will hit you way harder than a regular rum and cola. Sweet, right? So drink up—just make sure you're drinking the hard stuff straight or with diet mixers.

But you don't have to go so over-the-top with this stuff. Another great dieter drink? Tequila. Jose Cuervo Especial—both the Gold and Silver varieties—has 40 percent alcohol and is 65 calories per 1-ounce shot. That's awesome, provided you're willing to drink it the grownup way, with salt and lime. If you want that tequila turned into a 12-ounce margarita using Jose's mix, you're looking at over 400 calories. That's probably not going to work with your daily allotment.

Regardless of what they're distilled from, most traditional 80-proof hard liquors are in this range—around 65 calories per 1-ounce shot—so it doesn't really matter whether you prefer vodka, Scotch, bourbon, gin, or rum. What does matter is what you mix it with. Every bar and bartender has a different way of pouring and mixing a drink, so it's hard to know exactly what you're getting when you order, say, a martini or a whiskey sour. It's up to you to ask for exactly what you want and make sure you get it.

🍷🍸 Liquor

SMART

Rum and Diet Coke	140 calories
2 shots rum and diet soda	
Mojito	150 calories
2 ounces rum, 1 ounce lime juice, two sprigs fresh mint, 1 packet Splenda, Sweet'N Low, or Equal, and soda water	
Skinny Greyhound	150 calories
Diet grapefruit soda or Squirt plus 2 shots gin	

STUPID

Jagerbomb	215 calories
Half a can of Red Bull and 1 shot Jagermeister	
(If you're in the mood for a Jagerbomb, use Sugar Free Red Bull, which would still be 120 calories.)	

Remember that sweet, fruity stuff adds up quickly, and there are calories in tonic water—it may not taste like it, but there's sugar in there. My advice? If you prefer mixed drinks, identify the possible light variations on the drinks you like and ask the bartender to cut out anything you can pass on.

In other words, ask for that martini dry. Extra, super, Phoenix-in-a-drought dry. Two ounces of Tanqueray gin is around 150 calories. That kiss of dry vermouth will cost you about 10 calories—there are 55 calories in an ounce of the stuff, so watch what the bartender puts in and note accordingly. The olive is about 5 calories, depending on its size. That means you've got about 165 calories in that glass, provided you get a real martini, not some newfangled sour apple thing loosely based on a recipe from *Sex and the City*. As I said, it's time to put on your grownup pants.

Liqueurs and Alcopops

On the other side of the spectrum, you find stuff like Baileys Irish Cream and Parrot Bay Caribbean Coconut Rum. Parrot Bay has about 70 calories per ounce, just like real rum, but only half as much alcohol. Bummer. Likewise, it shouldn't surprise you that the liqueurs like Baileys and Kahlúa are calorie-killers. Those syrupy sweet concoctions are like spiked milk shakes when it comes to calories. A regular white Russian with four shots of Kahlúa, two shots of vodka, and 3 ounces of whole milk comes in at a bowling-ball-heavy 736 calories.

Schnapps? Triple sec? Chambord? Amaretto? Forget about them; they're dead to you.

Likewise, alcopops like Zima (231 calories), Smirnoff Ice (248 calories), and Sparks (257 calories) should be avoided at all costs. Ditto for the light versions—Mike's Lite Hard

Lemonade, for example, has only 3.2 percent alcohol and 100 calories.

If you just can't live without sweetness in your drink, consider adding fruit juices to liquor, which more or less gives the same fruity flavor you'd get from, say, Sour Apple Pucker schnapps (72 calories per ounce, 15 percent) without all the calories. Orange juice, for example, has about 80 calories per 6-ounce serving, so mixed with 2 ounces of vodka to make a screwdriver, you're at 220 calories. Not good, but not terrible. Lemon juice has only about 20 calories per ounce, so a 2-ounce vodka-lemon, which isn't totally unlike a margarita, is only about 100 calories.

♟🍸 Try the Big Chubowski

This mixed drink has only about 160 calories. Make it with 2 shots vodka, ½ cup chilled coffee, and 2 teaspoons nondairy creamer. Combine ingredients, stir, and pour over crushed ice.

Wine

Unlike beer, wine benefits from fairly rigid standards among styles. That is to say, one wine maker's Burgundy is pretty much the same as the next, at least when it comes to calories. That makes things easy-peasy for dieters. No need to track down nutrition info in French or convert it from kilojoules!

Overall, the caloric differences between varieties of wine varies much less than those of beer or liquor, too. Probably because there are only two ingredients: grapes and yeast. Furthermore, most wines are pretty good calorie bargains.

Bordeaux, Cabernet Sauvignons, Chiantis, Sauvignon Blancs, Merlots, Zinfandels, Rieslings, and other common wines come in around or just under 100 calories per 4-ounce glass and are typically between 12 and 15 percent alcohol.

White wines actually tend to be a little better on the calorie-to-alcohol front than red wines, but not by any appreciable margin and with many exceptions. And, of course, we've been hearing for years how drinking a glass of red wine every day is great for our health (it packs lots of antioxidants, procyanidins, and resveratrol), so let's go ahead and assume all that science is semi-sound. That makes a glass of red a pretty nice companion to your frozen dinner, provided you have someone to share the bottle with. If you don't have someone to share a bottle with, avoid ordering one out—even if you drink three glasses of wine over a few hours and it would have been cheaper to buy a bottle and get the fourth for free. If you've got a whole bottle, you're quite likely to end up overindulging to finish it, which isn't good, since a typical 750-milliliter bottle of wine has between 350 and 500 calories in it. That means drinking the whole thing is a big calorie commitment for most dieters.

It's a much better idea to go the boxed—ahem, *cask*—wine route. Luckily, in addition to being, shall we say, a bit more modestly priced, boxed wine makes portion control easy. Twist open the spout, pour a serving, and seal it back up. If you get a 5-liter box—er, *cask*—you'll be able to pour almost exactly one month's worth of daily 5-ounce servings out of it. That's just about how long it lasts before the taste starts to deteriorate, too. A month of daily drinks for $12? Not bad!

Still not sold? Well, boxed wines are consistently improving as more and more wineries jump on board, but I think a guilt trip would be a better way to convince you. Boxed wine is also much, much better for the environment. As the *New York Times* has reported, switching from bottles to boxes cuts wine's carbon footprint in half. That means that if California wineries switched the packaging of the wine they ship back east from bottles to boxes, they'd save about 2 million tons of carbon dioxide in shipping per year. That's the equivalent of retiring 400,000 cars. Or like putting every single resident of Raleigh, North Carolina, on a bicycle.

Since 97 percent of wines are made to be consumed within a year, buying wine in vessels made to last about that long makes a lot of sense. The old ideas about boxed wine being déclassé come exclusively from outmoded ideas Americans have about aging fine European wines in cellars. Most people don't do that and, if they do, they have no right to judge you while you're in line at the supermarket anyway. If they're *so* classy that they only drink fancy-ass wine *with a cork in it,* shouldn't their butler be out doing the shopping? So buy the boxed wine because it's best for both your diet and Mother Earth. And if anyone gives you any shit, haughtily tell them they're killing the ozone and that they should be ashamed of themselves. Works every time.

♀⚱♀ Wine

SMART

Franzia Merlot	105 calories per 5 ounces	12.5% alcohol
Dom Perignon	110 calories per 5 ounces	12.5% alcohol

STUPID

Arbor Mist White Zinfandel Exotic Fruit		
	105 calories per 5 ounces	6% alcohol

Just in case you need another little nudge, mass-market boxed wines tend to be a little lighter than their fancy bottled counterparts. Franzia—the world's most popular wine, or so the company claims—sells some of the lightest wines you'll find. The highest calorie count of anything they make—and they make Cabs, Zins, blushes, Merlots, Chiantis, and pretty much everything else—is 110 calories per 5-ounce serving. The lowest, Refreshing White, is only 90 calories per 5-ounce serving. Anyone can budget that into their daily allotment.

It's not all blissful in grapeland, though. Ice wines, dessert wines, and sangria are better off avoided. A full-size glass of muscatel can set you back 160 calories, and ports are even worse. So be sure to steer clear of the supersweet stuff that comes in those expensive mini-bottles—you want the regular stuff. In a box, please.

Cannabis

The following is a post from an Internet forum catering to cannabis users, written by someone who calls himself "Hippie John":

> I was thinking, since marijuana gives you the munchies, its probably becasue of higher metabolizm, thus making you hungry. But think if you didnt eat anything even when you were really really hungry? The high metabolizm would burn off fat like you wouldnt beleive.

In addition to a few minor spelling errors in his well-reasoned piece, Hippie John doesn't seem to have much of an understanding of marijuana's influence on "metabolizm." Then again, neither does anyone else. For obvious reasons, the actual effect of marijuana on your body's rate of processing energy hasn't been studied much. It's hard enough to get the government to support marijuana studies involving cancer and AIDS patients, I guess, without bringing the comparatively trivial matter of weight loss into play.

There is, however, one thing we know for sure: Smoke contains no calories. Maybe marijuana increases your metabolism slightly, maybe it decreases it slightly, but, either way, it's not actually putting any food into your belly. Not directly, anyway.

There is, however, the phenomenon known as "the munchies." It's a rumored side effect of cannabis use whispered about among conclaves of our society's outcasts and in seedy drug dens. Anyway, druggies, dropouts, and the other sorts of lowlife that use this dangerous and illegal drug claim smoking marijuana will increase appetite. Who'd believe anything those filthy hippies have to say, though, right?

On the other hand, despite what *Reefer Madness*–minded puritans believe, marijuana doesn't actually make it impossible to control your behavior. Well, unless it's BC bud taken directly from Marc Emery's personal stash, in which case all bets are off. But if you've got regular cheap Mexican weed, you're totally capable of smoking a bowl and not eating a bag of Funyuns.

Yes, you are.

Shut up.

It's a willpower thing. Maybe you could eat a bowl of popcorn or a salad instead? Maybe you could just not eat anything? Either way, while it might not "burn off fat like you wouldnt beleive," as our friend Hippie John hypothesizes, smoking marijuana will cause a pleasant, borderline-euphoric sensation without costing you a single calorie.

Just steer clear of the pot brownies. A tiny 2-inch square

♀🍷🍸 **What you can drink for less than 200 calories?**

Here are six options, broken down by how much intoxicating ethanol each has.

Three shots (3 ounces) Smirnoff Red Vodka. You'll get 1.2 ounces of ethanol.

Two glasses (8 ounces) Carlo Rossi Burgundy. You'll get 1.08 ounces of ethanol.

Two bottles Miller Lite. You'll get 1 ounce of ethanol.

One bottle Hornsby's Hard Cider. You'll get .66 ounce of ethanol.

Two shots (2 ounces) Sour Apple Pucker. You'll get .3 ounce of ethanol.

One (1.5 ounces) Buttery Nipple shot. You'll get .2 ounce of ethanol.

---

of most brownie recipes has over 200 calories. And, of course, the effect of ingested marijuana lasts a lot longer than the effect of smoked marijuana, making it necessary to control your appetite longer. And once you've got the taste of chocolate in your mouth, things can get fuzzy. Maybe you can make it without eating anything other than a 2-inch square of brownie, maybe you can't, but it's better not to risk it.

HOW TO WORK OUT (WITHOUT LOOKING LIKE A TOOL)

We are underexercised as a nation. We look instead of play. We ride instead of walk. Our existence deprives us of the minimum of physical activity essential for healthy living.
—JOHN F. KENNEDY

I HAVE NEVER STEPPED FOOT IN A GYM OR HEALTH CLUB. NOT since my college racquetball class, anyway. *It's just not my scene, man.*

Now, I know plenty of cool people go to the gym, and I'm sure there are even a few health clubs across the country that cater specifically to hip young people, but I still consider them douchey dens of spray-tanned meatheads and tacky women dressed like Fergie. Forced to make small talk with some 'roid monkey in short shorts while waiting to sit on a sweaty machine? Holding my nose while standing around in the putrid stank of a stuffy locker room trying not to catch an eyeful of some old man's junk? Listening politely as some intense chick with short, spiky hair offers me pointers on my form?

No thanks.

I do, however, exercise three to five times a week. And so should you. You don't have to work out to lose weight, of course, but it certainly helps. We've talked a lot about how many calories your body burns sitting still and how many calories you ingest when you consume various foods, and it's obvious that you can control those numbers so the former is greater than the latter. Still, it's nice to get a little extra edge.

First, a big disclaimer: I don't eat more calories because I'm exercising and neither should you. It's too easy to end up taking an overly rosy view of how far you pushed yourself and cheat. If you're taking on some extreme challenge, like a marathon or an Ironman, then there's a bit of flexibility. But, generally, you should *not* adjust your calorie limit upward. Stick with the numbers you came up with earlier, even if you're running a 5K a few times a week. Just think of that workout as a little bonus boost and maybe a little cushion in case you underestimated some of the foods you ate. I know this sounds particularly extreme if you've looked at any iPhone apps—almost all of which seem to have a place to add exercise and raise your daily calorie target—but sticking to your original numbers is for the best.

People who count on exercise to lose weight usually fail, as science has shown. Just look at a study conducted by the Pennington Biomedical Research Center in Baton Rouge, Louisiana, comparing people who lost weight by cutting 25 percent of their calories and people who lost weight by cutting 12.5 percent of their calories and adding enough exercise to burn 12.5 percent more energy. To get the exercisers to the same level of loss as the calorie-cutters, they had to work out for a full hour every single day.

"In general, exercise by itself is pretty useless for weight loss," Professor Eric Ravussin, one of the academics behind the study, told the *New York Times*. "Take in fewer calories than you burn, put yourself in negative energy balance, lose weight."

Take in fewer calories than you burn . . . lose weight. Yes, that's yet another serious scientist preaching the simple strategy outlined here. You'd think every weight-loss book would say this stuff!

So, if we've established that working out doesn't earn you more food, you might be wondering what's in it for you. Aside from the fact that a lot of physical activities are actually sorta fun, there is evidence that exercise can help you keep weight off once you've lost it.

A study by the National Weight Control Registry found that about 90 percent of people who successfully maintained their weight loss worked out regularly. Of course, correlation does not imply causation—it's possible that people who were dedicated enough to work out were also dedicated enough to successfully limit their calories—but those numbers suggest to me that working out isn't a bad idea. We'll talk more about maintenance later, but that's something to keep in mind as you plan to incorporate physical activity into your day.

If you're inclined to buy a gym membership, you'll have a number of options. Classes, elliptical machines, lap pools—all sorts of stuff like that. If you're into such things, go ahead and skip to the next chapter now. No problemo. Some bro-dawg in a polo shirt can probably tell you a lot more about working out than I can. You guys can get protein shakes together and hang out talking about spandex and shit. Don't worry, you won't hurt my feelings. I'm just gonna be chillin' here, *not* mentioning anything about major muscle groups. No biggie, brah.

Always Take the Stairs

By now we've successfully established that (a) exercise is good but not a substitute for strict adherence to your calorie limit and (b) you don't need to go to the gym. Where does that leave you? Looking for ways to get a good little workout around the place we live, often without people even necessarily noticing we're in the process of doing it.

Seriously, the line between "sedentary" and "moderately active" is a very thin one. You can get your blood flowing and burn a few calories in the very simplest ways without even realizing it. How?

Always take the stairs. It's pretty easy to commit to never riding an elevator or escalator again. Help all your friends move when they ask—they'll love you for it. Volunteer to walk down to the coffee shop and get your colleagues their daily cuppa—you'll score huge points with everyone. Clean the shit out of your apartment every week—doing the windows requires nearly as much bending, flexing, and stretching as yoga with the added benefit of getting clean windows. Walk the dog until his little paws ache—dogs love that.

The important thing is to do something active. *Anything* active. Most tables of suggested calorie intake by age and gender tell people they can have about 200 more calories per day if they move from "sedentary" to "moderately active."

If you're already "moderately" active, you'll get a similar 200-calorie bump by going up to "very active." That doesn't sound like a lot, I know, but you're looking at nearly half a pound over the course of a week without doing anything that'll make you sore the next morning. That's a pretty sweet deal.

Whoever you are, wherever you live, there are definitely a few little things you can do.

Just think about it for a minute.

. . .

Got some ideas?

Great, now make a mental commitment to doing them.

Better yet, raise your right hand right now and repeat after me: I'll always take the stairs. And I'll also . . .

Maybe you want something a little more serious than that. If so, I applaud you. As I said, exercise isn't just a good way to promote weight loss, it's a great way to enjoy the lifestyle you're working for. When you're fat, it's hard to remember how rewarding strenuous physical activity can be, and maybe my very favorite part of the whole weight-loss experience was rediscovering my love of the outdoors.

Sounds a little sappy, I know, but it's totally true. During my diet, I took up walking, running, hiking, biking, and kayaking. I've since hiked up and down the Grand Canyon, along 20 miles of impossibly gorgeous alpine trail on New Zealand's Routeburn Track, and to the summit of California's Mount Whitney, the highest point in the Lower 48. Around home, I've enjoyed the simple pleasures of biking to the grocery store to buy frozen dinners and apples and kayaking the rivers and lakes of central Arizona. Oh, and I also ran a real race, the 5-mile Turkey Trot in Cleveland on an icy cold

Thanksgiving morning. I rounded the course—which took me by landmarks like the Rock and Roll Hall of Fame and Cleveland Browns Stadium—at just over 8 minutes a mile, a pace I was pretty proud of.

True, these are modest adventures in the grand scheme of things. I haven't done anything that required an ice ax or putting tape over my nipples. But I never, ever, would have been able to do any of these things at nearly 300 pounds, and they're things I really, *really* loved doing. And they're things I want you to do, too, if you're so inclined.

But let's start small.

Fidgeting (Until Someone Around You Snaps)

Fidgeting burns a significant number of calories. Really. So does pacing, tapping your toe, rocking your chair back and forth, and lots of other little nervous tics that annoy the shit out of everyone around you. They're all classified as non-exercise activity thermogenesis (NEAT), which is defined by a Mayo Clinic researcher as "the energy expended for everything we do that is not sleeping, eating, or sports-like exercise."

Dr. James Levine, an endocrinologist and professor of medicine at Mayo, studied NEAT by putting volunteer subjects in special underwear with sensors that tracked their smallest motions. In an article for *Science,* he reported that fidget-prone people burned an extra 350 calories a day.

Yes, that's a pound every two weeks for tapping your damn pencil all the fucking time while the people in the cubicle next to you just want to do their stupid work in peace and get home, asshole. I'm not suggesting you try to turn yourself into a fidgeter, necessarily, but if you've been fighting the urge, feel free to let 'er loose and reap the benefits.

Chewing Gum (Like a Cow Chews Her Cud)

Actually, that Dr. Levine is a little obsessive about this NEAT stuff. According to the *Los Angeles Times,* he has a treadmill at his desk so he can walk while he works and stay in perpetual motion. A small study of the "walk-and-work desk," a Levine-created contraption that a company is now selling for $4,500, even got published in the *British Journal of Sports Medicine.*

Also, Levine wrote a paper called "Interindividual Variation in Posture Allocation: Possible Role in Human Obesity," which, just as its name implies, compared the stance of lean and obese people using sensors. He discovered that obese people were seated, on average, two hours longer every day than their leaner counterparts. Interesting, right?

But maybe Levine's all-time best project was published as a letter to the *New England Journal of Medicine*—the oldest and most prestigious medical journal in the world, mind you. The letter, "The Energy Expended in Chewing Gum," cited serious gum-chewing research conducted "in a temperature-controlled, darkened, silent laboratory with an indirect calorimeter."

His conclusion?

"Gum chewing is sufficiently exothermic that if a person chewed gum during waking hours and changed no other components of energy balance, a yearly loss of more than 5 kg of body fat might be anticipated. Chewing of calorie-free gum can be readily carried out throughout the day, and its potential effect on energy balance should not be discounted."

By the way, 5 kilograms is about 11 pounds, which is not a trivial number at all. *Just for chewing gum all day.* If you're one of those people who can walk *and* chew gum, well, this weight-loss thing should be a snap.

Standing (at a Concert)

Different studies show that most people burn between 33 and 50 percent more calories standing than they do sitting. For a 150-pound person, that could be 400 over the course of an eight-hour workday if you can get your boss to spring for one of those nifty stand-up desks.

Otherwise, stand on your own time. You would probably burn 200 calories over the course of a four-hour concert. Not bad, right? So stand for the show—it's more rock 'n' roll, anyway—and make your body do a little extra work.

Walking (Whenever You Can)

Many of the brightest minds in human history were big walkers. Thoreau said people didn't believe him when he told them he tended to "walk every day about half the daylight." Thomas Jefferson, on the other hand, limited himself to only two hours of walking a day.

Emerson, Kierkegaard, Dickens, and Twain were all hard-core walkers. Want a longer list? Turns out a minister from Cuyahoga Falls, Ohio, a town next to the one where I grew up, actually wrote a book profiling the habits of fifty famous walkers, including Gandhi, Martin Luther King Jr., Carl Jung, César Chávez, and C. S. Lewis. He argues that walking brings about "physical, mental, and spiritual renewal," and I'm not inclined to disagree.

In fact, when it comes to walking, the minister is in agreement with the man who proclaimed God dead. Friedrich Nietzsche declared, "All truly great thoughts are conceived while walking."

Walking is also a solid exercise option. The number of

calories you burn walking depends greatly on how fast you do it and how large you are to begin with, but it's always an easy, low-impact way to go. Also, it doesn't really look as if you're in the middle of a sweaty workout, so you can get some exercise in while wearing jeans, leaving the people you pass to think you're simply in a hurry to get somewhere and cannot afford a car or bike. Depending on where you live, you may walk a bit already. That's great. Now walk more. How close is the grocery store to your house? What about work? Surely there has to be someplace you can hoof it, even if it's just some park down the street where teenagers congregate to illicitly smoke cigarettes, engage in sexting, and trade blowjays for jelly bracelets. Or whatever it is kids are up to nowadays.

Despite what you'll read around the interwebs, the energy expenditure for walking and running the same distance is *not* the same. Sorry, the old "your body is moving the same distance so it's using the same fuel" logic just doesn't cut it. Researchers at Syracuse University studied this in 2004 and found that people burn about twice as many calories running a mile as walking a mile, on both a track and a treadmill. Still, walking is a lot easier on your joints and doesn't necessarily require an extra shower afterward, so it's not a big deal to work into your day.

You want some sort of quantification, don't you? Well, the calories you burn while walking or running are largely a function of how efficient your stride is. You'll find all sorts of numerical values assigned to particular exercises, but they're the product of research done on people with different arms and legs and who move differently than you do, so take them with a grain of salt. But, based on the above-mentioned study, you can expect to burn somewhere between 40 and 100 calories for every mile you walk. That'll certainly help—as long as you don't add it to your food allotment.

Running (Shoes Matter)

As outlined above, jogging burns about twice as many calories per mile as walking. Depending on your gender, size, and pace, you're looking at somewhere around 100 calories per mile. Personally, I love running, but I know a lot of people who've had major problems because of it, suffering debilitating injuries that short-circuited their fitness regimes for months and months.

If you want to run after a long period of inactivity, you need to start slowly, strengthening your muscles and limbering up your joints, before you get too crazy with things.

You also need to be careful about shoes. That's true for any runner, but especially, I believe, for people who are carrying a few extra pounds. I discovered this myself the hard way.

My first running shoes came from Goodwill, a pair of more-than-slightly-worn Asics that cost me $5 and worked really well. I was running 3 miles a few times a week with no problems. Then I outsmarted myself and made an upgrade, buying a pair of higher-end Sauconys with the standard high-rise heel to help cushion my steps. Big mistake. Within a few weeks, both my back and the metatarsals in my feet were aching.

Here's what I discovered: Shoes really matter when running, and the best running shoes for some people may be the least-cushioned ones.

This thinking is in line with the barefoot running movement, one of the huge trends in the sport at the moment. There's an excellent book all about barefoot running, Christopher McDougall's *Born to Run,* and I've been assured by friends, family, and my girlfriend that my proselytizing on McDougall's behalf is superannoying. So I'll try to keep it short, and I'll spare you a lecture about the awesome Tarahumara Indians in Mexico. *Sigh.*

The gist of the barefoot argument is this: Modern running shoes greatly alter our natural stride, which can lead to injuries. Our feet and legs are naturally very efficient at absorbing the shock of landing when we run, but superstructured running shoes add a massive amount of cushion under the heel, making us pervert our stride by allowing us to land on our heels instead of the front of our foot, where we would naturally fall. The foam on the shoe absorbs a lot of the shock, of course, but not all of it, and the extra impact ends up traveling through our knees and hips into our lower back, leading to serious injury.

This is why, as a recent article in *Sports Science* pointed out, more people get injured running, despite all the "advances" in modern shoe technology.

Here's how Harvard professor Daniel E. Lieberman put it in a news release that accompanied a study he did on barefoot running for the journal *Nature:*

People who don't wear shoes when they run have an astonishingly different strike. By landing on the middle or front of the foot, barefoot runners have almost no impact collision, much less than most shod runners generate when they heel-strike. Most people today think barefoot running is dangerous and hurts, but actually you can run barefoot on the world's hardest surfaces without the slightest discomfort and pain. All you need is a few calluses to avoid roughing up the skin of the foot.

This is something every runner should consider, but since you're overweight, it's even more important. Think about it: You may be dropping twice as much weight on your heels as a typically twiggy runner. Your knees, legs, and back are not twice as strong. Understandably, that could lead to some problems.

This is, I think, why those shoes with the raised heel messed me up. The Goodwill shoes were pretty much beat, having already been used until the foam lost most of its support, meaning I wasn't overrelying on the heel. The brand-new pair encouraged me to heel-strike, and I started hurting. So I ended up buying a pair of Nike Free Run shoes. Hardcore barefooters would laugh and say they're not "barefoot enough," but I like them, although I later got a pair of Vibram FiveFingers and I like them, too. My advice is to go as natural as possible, trusting your body to adapt without an expensive piece of foam. Others disagree. A running store can test your stride for pronation, supination, and all that other stuff and make professional recommendations about your footwear.

Hiking (Yeah, It's a Lot Like Walking)

Yes, hiking is a lot like walking—but with mud, pointy rocks, beautiful scenery, and maybe an animal or two if you're lucky. It's also, in my opinion, the very best exercise you can do.

It's pretty hard to quantify a lot of the benefits of hiking—feeling connected to the natural world, the sense of peace that comes from getting off the grid, the fresh air of the forest—but researchers have tried. In fact, in 2007 the University of Essex conducted a study on depressed people, having them walk either through the woods and on a trail

---

🥿 Calories Burned During Various Activities You May or May Not Do from Time to Time

These figures are per hour for a 150-pound person. Add or subtract for someone heavier or lighter.

Bowling in an ironic hipster bowling league: 216
Doing a twist dance like Uma Thurman in *Pulp Fiction:* 432
Watching *Mad Men:* 81
Kayaking: 360
Bicycling late to work at 20 mph: 1,188
Bicycling back home from the bar at 12 mph: 576
Moving apartments: 504
Raking your mother's lawn: 288
Skateboarding: 360
Doing Hatha yoga: 288
Golfing with your boss and carrying the clubs: 396

---

around a lake or in an indoor shopping mall. Not surprisingly, they found that walking in the woods reduced depression. Perhaps a little surprisingly, walking in a shopping center actually *increased* their depression.

The numbers weren't even close: 71 percent of participants said their depression decreased after hiking, while 22 percent said it increased after walking through the mall. A full 90 percent reported feeling a bump in their self-esteem after the hike, while 44 percent said they felt worse about themselves after walking around the shopping center. That's right, walking around a mall can actually make sad people sadder. Yikes.

Not that you're necessarily depressed, of course. Still, who couldn't stand to be a little happier? Hiking can do that for you, along with giving you a great workout. It's easy to find trails that'll push you as hard as a 40-minute jog without all the jarring motion.

The calories burned hiking depend on how steep and challenging the terrain you're crossing is and what you're carrying. It'd be too hard to get into all the various metrics at play here, but a 150-pound person could burn as many calories hiking 10 miles and gaining 4,500 feet in elevation as running a half marathon. And then there's backpacking, where you carry camping supplies with you in a pack probably weighing somewhere between 15 and 40 pounds. If you're backpacking, it's like being fat again, but in a good way: you're burning tons of extra calories because you're carrying extra weight!

A trail's distance is important, but the vertical gain is more important for cardio—a nice steep trail is a stair climber instead of a treadmill. I look for trails with a vertical rise of 1,000 feet in 1 mile. That takes me just under half an hour to complete, and I burn about 300 calories doing it. Then I walk down slowly. When a trail is that steep, it can actually be an intense aerobic workout, too, since my heart rate gets up near capacity when I really push myself. Depending on your weight, you're probably burning somewhere between 300 and 600 calories by hiking up 1,000 feet in 1 mile, which is about a 20 percent gradient and is the steepest you'll find in most city park systems.

Maybe you don't have any hills that big and steep where you live, in which case you'll find the biggest, steepest hill you can and do it as many times as it takes to get to 1,000 feet. Aim for the longest hill you can find with a 20-plus percent grade. Actually, that might be better than my preferred trails, since the breaks between uphill sprints would make it more like interval training. Serious athletes use interval training—alternating between pushing yourself as hard as you can and cooling down—to build endurance, and several studies have shown that it burns fat better than exercise at a consistent pace.

Biking (Cool and Practical)

Biking is "in" right now—whether it's spinning classes or fixies—and with good reason. First, actual biking is a practical way to get around. If there's a better way to make sure you exercise than to depend on it for transportation, I can't imagine what it is.

Even if you're not ready to take the leap and sell your car, you can still incorporate a bicycle into your life by using it for routine errands. I like to bike to the grocery store about a mile from my house and to meet friends for lunch at the pizza place across the street from the store. I've also found it's a great way to enjoy the paths along the canals in Phoenix.

The other big advantage of bicycling is that it's a low-impact aerobic activity. Like swimming—which requires a pool and isn't used as a mode of transportation anywhere I'm aware of—it's a fluid movement for your body that doesn't strain your joints. How many calories will you burn? That depends on how hard you pedal, how much you weigh, and the efficiency of your bike's gears. On the low end, a leisurely ride by a small rider on an efficient bike would burn only about 200 calories per hour. On the high end, a large person pedaling hard up hills on a simple one-gear bike could burn 1,000 calories or more per hour.

My advice: Go where you want to go and just enjoy the ride. After all, half the fun with biking is looking cool. Bikes are essential to the hipster experience right now—the hipster zeitgeist is seemingly inseparable from his wheels. Almost any crude Internet cartoon satirizing hipsters will feature a guy with facial hair and a fixed-gear bicycle. Urban Outfitters has even opened its own bike shop, if you can believe it. Biking is cool—and fits with your new lifestyle quite nicely.

Gaming (Because You Like Staring at a Screen)

Are you mildly agoraphobic? Reluctant to do anything that looks like exercise in front of other sentient beings? Maybe you just like to see yourself as a cartoon when you work out.

If so, there is another option: video games.

Nintendo pretty much invented the concept of active gaming with the Power Pad in 1988, and they brought it into the modern era with the Wii. They're still the leaders with *Wii Fit,* which is the third-highest-selling game not packaged with a new gaming console in gaming history (the top two are also Wii titles, *Wii Play* and *Mario Kart Wii*), but Sony and Microsoft both jumped in with their own active gaming before Christmas 2010. Trends change, but right now the future looks pretty bright for video games that require moving more than your thumb.

Can it help you lose weight? Studies say yes—if you do it regularly.

A University of Mississippi professor of health and exercise science conducted a study in which he gave a Wii to eight families for six months to see if it improved their fitness. During the first six weeks the families had the game, it was used on average for 22 minutes a day. The family's children got slightly more aerobically fit. Their activity dropped precipitously to only 4 minutes a day during the second six weeks, and the fitness improvements tailed off to nothing.

While a suspicious British consumer group's study pointed

🔲 Question: What should you wear when you work out?

Answer: For the most part, that's totally up to you. Maybe you prefer American Apparel's shiny workout shorts and some retro tube socks. Maybe you'd rather style out with some neon sweatbands and vintage track pants. Whatevs.

There's only one element of workout fashion that's high stakes, and that's your shoes. You're looking for something that provides the right fit and structure, preferably something that leaves the muscles in your feet free to move in a natural way. Luckily, the coolest vintage shoes are also some of the best for your feet, so you're not going to have to sacrifice form for function if you don't want to. Here are some suggestions, both modern and retro.

New Balance Retro Running Line
$55–150 FROM NEWBALANCE.COM

Pros: New Balance makes an entire line of retro running shoes that have varied levels of support but a consistently awesome throwback look. Generally, in the New Balance world higher model numbers denote more expensive and cushioned shoes. The $150 supercushioned NB 2000 is a retro style that should cradle weaker feet; I've owned two pairs of NB 574s—they come in both men's and women's sizes—that served me well. They come in a rainbow of colors and have a moderate level of support along with a nice big toe box so your toes can spread naturally.

Cons: New Balance is justifiably maligned as old man shoes. They go really well with the grampy chic Rivers Cuomo look—khaki slacks and a button-down shirt—but if that's not what you're looking for, you should steer clear.

continued on page 175

out that *Wii Fit* burns fewer calories than traditional house-
hold chores like washing dishes and vacuuming during a
10-minute span, a survey by the American Heart Association suggests these games actually encourage people to make
real-life fitness goals. They called it a "gateway" to exercise.

The AHA talked to 2,284 men and women between the
ages of twenty-five and fifty-five and found that 58 percent
of the people who play "active-play" video games decided to
move on to activities like jogging, walking, and tennis, with
68 percent reporting that they had become more physically
active since they started the games.

So start playing—at least until you decide to burn some
serious calories by washing the damned dishes.

Workout DVDs (They're Not Super Cool— But No One Will Know)

There is really nothing at all cool about aerobics classes—
except maybe the retro fashionable spandex and bumpin'
hip-hop beats. The workout routines you encounter in such
classes can, however, be an effective way to simultaneously
increase muscle strength and do a little cardio. Luckily, the
VCR made it unnecessary to attend class in a gym, and now
a vast array of workout routines are available on DVD, so you
can get the exact same workout taking recorded "classes" in
the comfort and safety of your own home. Magical!

I've done a few home workout DVDs and really enjoyed
the experience. It's good to measure yourself against the su-
perfit instructors, and you'll definitely wear out muscles you
forgot you had. It's also about the fastest workout you can
get. There's no travel time, obviously. Most of these videos
are calculated to really push you for 20 to 30 hard min-

continued from page 173

Nike Air Pegasus 89
$90 FROM NIKE.COM

Pros: Nike's Air Pegasus, named for a mythical winged horse, is the forerunner of many shoes in the company's current line. They're still updating this shoe, but this one is a reproduction of the original from 1989. It's supercushioned with a giant heel some people swear by.

Cons: Beware, you're probably gonna heel-strike in these.

KangaROOS Combat
$50 FROM ZAPPOS.COM

Pros: These are the original shoes with pockets that debuted in 1979, so they've got a great look and are minimalist-friendly. They're made of thin nylon, so they're not pulling your foot into an unnatural position, and they've also got a roomy toe box that mirrors the shape of most feet and hard foam that's too stiff to cushion your foot in an undesirable way.

Cons: Not real vintage. Also, you look like you're trying really hard.

Vibram FiveFingers
$75 FROM REI

Pros: They're very popular with barefoot running enthusiasts, who believe them to be a nice compromise between actually being barefoot and having a layer of protection to keep out the sharp and hard artifacts of our modern world.

Cons: They look superfruity and draw tons of attention, making it hard to work out in peace. However, I have a pair and really enjoy them—so long as I'm not out in a public park with lots of looky-loos.

continued on page 177

utes, then send you off to the showers. Just beware of any program that wants to sell you stupid crap you don't need (read: blow-up yoga balls) or pushes a dietary regiment that conflicts with this one (read: Atkins acolytes), but otherwise almost any will do.

This is not the time to go "indie" and try to discover an obscure up-and-comer. It's not like music—no one will be impressed that you were way ahead of the curve in embracing an exercise video "before it was cool." But if you are doing a workout video, trust the wisdom of the masses. I go with the famous names—Billy Blanks, Denise Austin, Amy Bento—and buy the videos that have top user ratings on Amazon.com, figuring the big-time franchises are most closely vetted by both experts and users.

Jillian Michaels' 30 Day Shred really kicked my ass, so I'm prepared to endorse it specifically. Watching the current queen of the workout video, who even has a boxed set on the shelves, bark at people on *The Biggest Loser* is pretty annoying. But it turns out that Jillian is great when she's *your* instructor. Just make sure you start with lighter hand weights and work your way up instead of trying to go whole hog and start with 12-pounders. It's also a good idea to keep a mirror nearby so you can be assured you're using proper form.

Weight Training (Just a Little)

Chances are you have very little interest in "getting swole" with a hardcore weightlifting regimen—such aspirations don't generally fit this book's aesthetic. However, increasing your muscle strength a bit does make a big difference in how you look and feel. It also helps strengthen your bones as well as your muscles, which decreases your risk of injuring yourself doing something else, so it's something you should *continued from page 175*

Nike Free Run
$85 FROM DICK'S SPORTING GOODS

Pros: They look like normal running shoes. They've got a lot more cushion than the extreme barefoot-style shoes.

Cons: Serious barefoot runners will tell you the heel on these things is way too big to fully realize the benefits of unshod running. They're the product of a huge, evil multinational corporation and possibly made in a Chinese sweatshop. Several pennies from the pair you buy may find their way into LeBron James's pockets, which is a good reason not to buy anything made by Nike.

Puma Speed Cat
$50 FROM FOOT LOCKER

Pros: Like the Roos, these vintage-style sneakers—originally made for wear during motorsports—look cool enough to wear out to a bar but have an incredibly thin sole, giving them a barefoot-like feel.

Cons: Kinda flashy-looking. Guilt by association: Perhaps no sport is douchier than motorcycle racing, and motorcycle racers often wear these.

Converse All Star
$30 FROM KOHL'S

Pros: The original original athletic shoe, they've got very little padding or support. Fashion-wise, they're as close to "classic" as anything in the typical hipster closet.

Cons: There's probably not enough padding to allow you to heel-strike in a big way, but because they're fairly narrow and the rubber on the sole is fairly stiff, your foot will not move as naturally as in other barefoot-style shoes. They do look cool, though, and are certainly better than a pair of modern, high-heel running shoes.

definitely look into. And know that it's something *you abso-lutely don't need to do on machines at the gym.* Yup, those giant metal contraptions are just idiotproof ways to do the same workouts you can do with simple free weights. I could try to describe a full free-weight strength training regimen in excruciating detail, but I've found that YouTube videos are worth easily 1,000 words.

You're looking for the classics — crunches, dumbbell squats, push-ups, bicep curls, chest flies, dumbbell rows, etc. It's incredibly important to make sure your form is correct with these exercises, since wasting your time is the best pos-sible outcome of doing them wrong. Catastrophic injury is another possibility. This actually might be the time to break down and hire a professional to show you the basics. You can then progress through the routine on your own, gradually increasing the amount of weight you lift as you get stronger. You can find a trainer at the gym or turn to a friend who is a personal trainer or has been going to a trainer long enough to know the drill by heart.

My advice: Find some videos that demonstrate the basics and try to learn as much as you can on your own without risking injury (ChubsterTheBook.com has the basic videos). Then, when you think you know what you're doing, find an expert to go through them with you and point out any prob-lems with your form. Then retreat to the privacy of your home and build those muscles up.

LOSING GRACEFULLY

When we lose twenty pounds, we may be losing the twenty best pounds we have! We may be losing the pounds that contain our genius, our humanity, our love and honesty.
—WOODY ALLEN

YOU'RE GOING TO BE ANNOYING WHILE YOU'RE ON THIS DIET. I'm warning you about that now.

You, in turn, should try to subtly warn the people who are forced to deal with you every day, either by choice or circumstance. I'm sorry to say this, but it's pretty much unavoidable. Maybe you'll be mildly agitating, maybe you'll be downright insufferable, but you're definitely going to be a pain in the ass at times.

This isn't something a lot of diet books talk about. That's probably because the net effect of dieting is so overwhelmingly good. Not just on the health front, but socially and psychologically, too. Studies have shown that people's lives usually improve after they lose weight. They're generally happier and have a better self-image, and their relationships, so long as they were generally happy before the diet, get better. Getting there is not always a picnic, though, and we're going to address the challenges because the whole point of Chubster is to lose weight without losing your cool.

Hunger leads to irritability, establishing new habits requires rigid discipline, and self-control means being a little self-absorbed. None of that's an excuse, though. You're going to be feeling better about yourself, and that will help offset things, but be aware that you're likely to be less than wonderful at some points. So here are a few things to keep in mind when you're trying not to alienate the people who care about you. (By the way, as should be obvious, these are all things I was guilty of myself, so I definitely understand how they can happen.)

Don't Be Too Crazy About Your Meal Schedule

When you're on a diet, sometimes, you're going to be hungry. That's a given. To combat that, I tend to eat small snacks throughout the day, never going more than three or four hours before I eat a little something.

This is not normal, however, and you can't expect everyone to stay on your schedule. Do what you can to have a little snack—pack an apple in your purse, keep some rice cakes under the seat of your car, fill your belly with hot coffee or tea when you can—but don't expect everyone to center their life around your snacking schedule.

Really, there's no reason to stress out or get irked by small things like the timing of food consumption. As we discussed a while back, despite what you've probably heard elsewhere, your metabolism is not actually increased substantially by eating frequent small meals. You could eat all 2,000 calories of your government-recommended diet in one sitting and be in pretty much the same spot. Unless you're already diabetic, your blood sugar is probably not spiking and splattering too violently, either. The only thing you're actually battling is hunger-induced crankiness, and it's your responsibility to battle that for the good of your fellow man. Just suck it up and smile until you're in a position to eat.

This starts with recognizing the source of your foul mood. If you feel yourself starting to get cranky while your appetite increases, try to remember that the simmering irritation is probably just the hunger talking and that you have perhaps not actually been aggrieved in a major way. Then try to have a little snack. If that's not possible, just stay calm and remember you'll be eating soon and that whining is unlikely to make that happen much sooner.

Don't Take Your Activity Time out of Your Social Time

Like any big change, dieting is going to alter your social scene a bit. It won't necessarily be a sea change, but it will affect things somehow. How much is largely up to you.

If, like me, you've got limited time for friends and hobbies, it's natural to try to combine the two. That works so long as your old friends are into your new hobbies. Sadly, not all of them will be.

I decided to follow my muse and dig deeper into my new interests. I quit my kickball league (kickball is sorta over, anyway) and spent my time on the trails. A lot of people from my old kickball team started doing the ironic bowling league thing; I bought a kayak. Not all of my friends were cool about my switching from "Sure, I'll be at happy hour" to "Hey, wanna go hiking tonight?" and I probably went further with it than I needed to, but that's what happens when you get new hobbies. So you make new friends who like your new hobbies. That's a little sad, sure, but that's how it works.

Still, you can do a lot to maintain your current friendships by making sure that you take your exercise time out of your personal time, not out of your time with others. Remember that not everyone is going to want to meet you at calorie-counting-friendly restaurants or go for a run. So go on their turf if you value those relationships and hope they try to meet you halfway down the road.

This goes for couples stuff, too. Hiking, I learned, does not count as a romantic date with your girlfriend if it's up a brutally steep hill in the middle of a hot summer day and ends with a trip to Subway. Whoops.

Be as Flexible as You Can About Where You Eat

While we've spent a lot of time going over what you can eat at various restaurants—establishing that you've pretty much always got a decent option—you've undoubtedly noticed that certain restaurants are a lot more diet-friendly than others. Likewise, it's hard to make sure you're properly appreciating things that are cooked for you at home. Some home-cooked meals are best enjoyed in a small portion before you go back for a second helping of salad—but it's the thought that counts.

You need to forget about all that. Or, at least, try not to let it rule your life. For example, there were a few weeks during my diet when I really wanted to eat only at Subway. The combination of all those fresh ingredients and ultralight calorie counts was intoxicating to me. Like Fogle before me, I wanted it for pretty much every meal. I was obsessed. Needless to say, this did not play well with everyone in my life, as normal people don't want one of twenty sandwiches—and, let's face it, they vary only slightly according to the meat involved—for every meal. So I had to compromise.

The point is this: Try your damnedest to be agreeable about where you eat when you eat with others. We've armed you with the knowledge to make the right picks anywhere, so don't be afraid to use it. It's easy to fall back on the old standbys, but it's not really cool, and it's not who you want to be. If it is, just put down this book and do Jared's plan.

Don't Preach

Preaching is generally bad in any context—whether you're talking to Madonna about teenage pregnancy or to a friend about the plate of saucy chicken wings in front of them at a bar.

This is going to feel unnatural, I know. If you're anything like me, you end up talking a lot about any big project you're working on or any totally amazing book you read (*ahem*). But with weight loss, things are a little different. The information you've acquired cries out for sharing—I know!—but people are touchy about weight- and food-related topics. Truthfully, if you're talking to your boss or a love interest, you're better off with a joke about the pope's engaging in an especially kinky sex act with Sarah Palin rather than trying to communicate the virtues and evils of various items on a chain restaurant menu. It almost never plays well.

Here's the thing: You and I know that no food is inherently

good or bad and that making responsible choices involves balancing desires and limits. You and I know what a calorie is and what our body will do with it. We're the enlightened few.

I find it genuinely fascinating that the body can do very different things with two Panda Express menu items that look and taste so much alike. So why not share that information? Yet I've been assured by a number of people that knowing such things "spoils" the meal for them. This isn't a "fat" or "skinny" thing, either. Some overweight people are totally comfortable discussing dieting in the abstract while some skinny people seem to feel judged. It's a weird dynamic, I know.

For me—and hopefully for you—calorie counts are interesting and inoffensive bits of trivia, much like a particular baseball player's slugging percentage. For others, what they eat is a deeply personal issue, often relating to their upbringing, and is possibly even politically charged. Comments that you mean to be innocuous and informative can come across as a major affront.

Much of America is either accidentally or willfully oblivious and happy to stay that way. We're not here to change them at this point—Congress will do that by mandating calorie counts on menus in the near future. If someone asks you a question, sure, tell them what they want to know. Maybe even suggest they buy a copy of a particular book you've enjoyed on the subject (*ahem*), but don't belabor the point. And whatever you do, don't initiate such conversations.

Tell Someone Who Cares

You're going to be pretty focused on dieting for the near future. That's good; you should be. Just remember that, like any hobby or interest, it has niche appeal. While as a whole your friends and family are likely to be quietly supportive— just watch for their eyes glazing over when you get into too many details—there are some people who truly find it fascinating. If you can find one of these people—sometimes they're overweight themselves, but just as often they find the whole idea of weight loss or gain fascinating because their weight stays mysteriously static regardless of what they eat—they'll be a great resource. They'll pepper you with questions, maybe ask for advice, and listen as you gripe about the little things that bother you about the Subway nearest your home.

If you have a significant other, this duty will probably fall to them. Take it from me, it's important not to go overboard. As happy as they may be to see you make a major life change, they're likely not quite as interested in it as you are. The important thing—or so I learned—is to make sure you're not any less interested in their goings-on. Asking how their day was *before* you bring up anything related to your calorie count is a great way to start.

Stupid Stuff People Say

As annoying as you may be to others while losing weight, some of them are going to annoy you right back. Usually not intentionally (not that it matters). A lot of people have no idea what sort of things are tactful to say to someone who is losing weight, and they'll often ask you unintentionally insulting questions or make dramatic compliments that actually sort of make you feel bad.

Did they think I was an ugly fat pig before I lost weight?
What, they didn't notice until now?
Why do they care how I did it?

Many people want desperately to encourage you. Odd as it may sound to a healthy and rational person, others might want to discourage you because of their own unconscious inferiority. Depending on how overweight you are, there may be people who were worried about you before but didn't know what to say. Other people might actually be trying to beat you down with what women's mags call "complisults." Either way, it's best to accept them graciously and then quickly change the subject.

Weight-loss compliments are a lot like condolences—the simpler, the better. As Dear Abby always says—and I'm paraphrasing here—the more you try to connect with someone about their dead grandma, the more likely you are to piss them off. The same goes for weight loss. Yet people try, so you need to be ready to handle it.

What they say: "You've lost some weight, haven't you. You're looking really good!"
What you're thinking: "Did I not look good before? Just how unattractive did you think I was before my weight loss?"
Unbiased interpretation: This is almost always a sincere compliment. Don't think too much about it; it's not backhanded. When someone says they like your shirt, do you worry they don't like any of your other shirts? Hopefully not, because that'd be crazy. Accept this graciously.
What you say: "Thanks!"

What they say: "It looks like you've lost some weight—what, about 20 pounds?"
What you're thinking: "Actually it's 46 pounds, asshole."
Unbiased interpretation: Most people have no ability whatsoever to accurately quantify weight loss. When they try, they

come across like a bad carnival barker manning one of those awful games with the giant scale. The guessing game isn't anything someone should do, but they probably don't realize how serious this process has been for you, and to them the guessing seems like a fun little game. So indulge them.

What you say: "Yup, that's right!"

What they say: "Wow, you're getting skinny! You're wasting away! Eat a cheeseburger!"

What you're thinking: "Ugh. I've still got 15 pounds to go before I'm at a normal weight—surely you can see that."

Unbiased interpretation: Some people really want to make some sort of remark about your weight loss but they're totally uncomfortable with it, so they go with the classic comic overstatement. People enjoy jokes, they assume, and it's hard to fault someone for saying you're *too* skinny. Little do they realize how much effort you've put into this and how much more you may have to go. Often people who drop this one on you are fat themselves, but it comes from all quarters, so try to just let it roll off your back.

What you say: "Ha-ha. Yeah!"

What they say: "Oh man, you're so much thinner now. You were pretty big before, almost as big as [insert shared acquaintance's name]!"

What you're thinking: "Ugh."

Unbiased interpretation: I cannot even count the number of people who've made fat jokes to me about other overweight people or about "the old Martin." I've never once found it even a little endearing. I'm not sure if skinny people always talk this way or if it's something they like to do with formerly obese people as a sort of bonding experience, but it's pretty terrible. As I said way back in the first chapter, I don't think there's necessarily anything wrong with being fat if you're willing to sacrifice the things you must to maintain that lifestyle. It's a poor choice, sure, but I'm not one to judge. *What you say:* "Yeeeeeeeah." (Be sure to drag the word out as long as possible—people will get the hint and change the topic without any sort of confrontation.)

What they say: "Wow, you've lost a lot of weight! What's your secret?"

What you're thinking: "No secret, asshole. I just counted calories. It was actually quite a bit of work."

Unbiased interpretation: With weight-loss surgery now being so common, any sort of dramatic weight loss is automatically suspicious to people. While certain medical maladies more or less require it, I'm generally wary of surgical solutions to weight problems, and I'm pretty sure you'll feel the same way after working hard to stick to your Chubster plan. They're dying to know how you did it, and they may be secretly hoping there's either some sort of trendy diet they can use themselves or, at the very least, a little juicy gossip. *What you say:* "Nope, just good old-fashioned diet and exercise!" (You may also want to toss in a little plug for this book . . . if it's not too much trouble.)

What they say: "Wow, you've lost a lot of weight. I respect that so much—I watch *The Biggest Loser* every week and I always cry!"

What you're thinking: "Oh my sweet Lord no. They think I'm like one of those pathetic losers on that stupid show! ARGH!"

Unbiased interpretation: I'm not sure there's anything that's given average-sized people a less realistic idea about weight loss than *The Biggest Loser*. I'm glad Jillian Michaels, Bob Harper, and the gang have done so much to inspire people, but the program *Loser* contestants participate in bears no resemblance to the one I did. I've only watched the show a few times, but it seems to me that it dramatically overemphasizes the role exercise plays while marginalizing the eating aspect. The contestants brutalize themselves in the gym so harshly, I have to imagine they eat a little more than they need to, and the results aren't quite what they could be with a more moderate, calorie-centric approach. Of course, footage of people *not* eating cupcakes doesn't make for much of a show, so they go the dramatic, over-the-top exercise route. Do people really think losing weight has to involve so much grunting and crying? Conversations I've had suggest so. *What you say:* "Yeah, a lot of people really like that show."

Keeping Your Momentum

Not all the psychosocial side effects of weight loss are negative, of course. You're going to feel pretty damn good about yourself. You can probably handle that feeling on your own for the most part, but here are a few ideas for staying motivated and enjoying your progress.

Get Your Thrift On

Having clothing that appears to fit you is key to not looking or feeling like a loser while you're dieting. Even if you've lost weight, you won't necessarily look or feel better when you're swimming in an oversized T-shirt and baggy jeans. So buy some new clothes. Nothing expensive—not until you're at your goal, anyway—but things that fit. I'm a big fan of thrift stores, as I'm sure you are.

As I shrunk out of my old clothes, I dropped them off at the back door of Goodwill—that's a good way to make sure you don't slip into old habits. Then I went back around front to find new stuff. It's amazing what you can find at Goodwill if you're willing to paw through a few musty old man shirts to dig up the gems. The looking, of course, is a big part of the fun. I spent an inordinate amount of time prowling the racks at every thrift store within driving distance of my house and was able to replace a lot of my wardrobe at ridiculously low prices. While I can't prove definitively that there is such a thing as "thrift store karma," I always found that when I gave away cherished or expensive items of clothing, I found great stuff in return—sometimes nearly the exact same thing in a smaller size.

I also made a habit of picking out shirts that were just a little too small for me every month or so, then looking forward to the day when I could slip them over my shoulders and have a nice cool new shirt to enjoy.

Time Your Goals to Special Events

Using the figures you came up with in the first chapter, you probably have a pretty good idea how fast you'll be dropping pounds. So don't be afraid to look ahead a few weeks or months and pick a nice round (pun not intended) number you'd like to hit by the next major holiday or special event. Got a wedding to attend in April? Set a goal. What about a pool party on the Fourth of July? Set a goal. Birthday in October? Yup, set a goal.

Perhaps you like to travel a bit, too. I found that trips made for even better motivation. Picturing the newly thinner version of myself swimming in the cool turquoise waters below Havasu Falls (Google it) or hiking along a trail through the southern Alps was a great motivator when I was lugging my ass up Squaw Peak in Phoenix on a summer day. And there was the first time I flew after losing weight, finally realizing that the seats weren't as tiny as I'd always thought they were and that it was actually possible to enjoy a few hours in the air. Wow. So look at a calendar and set some goals—it'll make the time slip by more quickly.

Keep Old Photos Handy

As you make progress, you're going to be amazed at how much your appearance changes. Seriously, people look a lot different when they lose weight! I get a comment every time I hand over my driver's license, and douchey near-campus bars have even double-carded me.

Your Facebook profile and the pictures on your bookshelf will tell you how far you've come, so relish them. The nice thing about Facebook photos is that they're already out there, so you don't need to risk coming across as an insufferable narcissist to show them to friends. Some people I've talked to also like to find a photo of themselves at their fattest and incorporate that into their routine somehow, maybe looking at it before they go out to eat or every morning when they get up. That seems a little extreme to me, but if you like the idea, go for it.

Visit Your Doctor

Nothing makes weight loss feel more official than having someone in a white jacket write that number on an important piece of paper. Chances are, your health insurance offers you one or two check-ups a year with a primary-care physician, so go ahead and take advantage of them. Schedule your next check-up for six months in the future before walking out the door, and you'll have a nice special event coming up to keep you on track. There's nothing like someone with a stethoscope putting you on a scale to make it seem serious.

Doctors scare people thin. *Permanently.* At least that's what it looks like based on a study that examined the effectiveness of weight-loss programs based on the events that triggered them. The article, "Long-term weight loss maintenance," in the *American Journal of Clinical Nutrition,* found that medical triggers were *the* most effective inducement to dieting, coming in ahead of things like "seeing a picture or reflection of themselves in the mirror."

Medical triggers were defined pretty loosely by researchers—everything from a doctor's warning to a relative's heart attack—and not only did they cause people to lose more weight, but they also increased the likelihood of their keeping it off. Unfortunately, there were no specific categories for "watching a diabetic amputee with a giant pepperoni grease stain rolled out of Pizza Hut in a wheelchair," "watching as a wall is knocked out so paramedics can pry an extremely fat neighbor out of her bed," and "taking naughty pictures for sexting but realizing you look too gross to send them." I suspect those experiences are even more effective, should you have the opportunity. Either way, medical scares are good motivation.

Doctors also usually know a little bit about dieting and exercising, so they can answer any questions you might have and maybe offer a few helpful suggestions. They're also generally huge supporters of weight loss, so they'll probably give you a few nice words of encouragement. Most primary-care physicians aren't superbusy with real shit—that's why they'll refer you to a specialist for anything more serious than a hangnail—and there's nothing they love better than giving people like you stern warnings.

Schedule a Test of Physical Prowess

As we've discussed, exercise isn't the best tool for losing weight, but your ability to enjoy rigorous physical activities is one of the major payoffs. It turns out that hiking, playing sports, and the like are actually kinda fun. You're going to be able to push yourself in ways you haven't in a long, long time, and that's a good thing.

So sign up for a race—anyone can run a 5K with a tiny bit of training, and a 10K or half marathon is easily within your grasp. Schedule a backpacking trip or a long group bike ride across town. Maybe look into a triathlon. Join a recreational sports league and set out to achieve a specific goal by the end of the season. What about walking to work every day for a month?

Whatever sort of exercise ends up winning you over, aim to do it better, longer, and faster. You'll find it helps keep you focused and inspired and provides another way of measuring your progress.

Plan a Special Post-Diet Meal

Since you're counting calories, you can technically have any food you want on any given day. Except gingerbread. But, of course, you're unlikely to do that because the tradeoff is going hungry the rest of the day, which is no fun. There's no such thing as a "cheat" day in Chubster, because you're cheating only yourself. What's the point in slowing down your progress by indulging in something silly?

Once you've hit your absolute final goal, however, you don't have to worry about "progress." So eat something decadent and *try* not to count it. After all the counting you've done, trying to set aside the concept of calories for one meal won't be easy, trust me, but it's important to allow yourself a little indulgence from time to time. Obviously, you can't do this every day after you finish your goal or you'll quickly be back at Chapter 1. But one decadent meal won't hurt—think of it as visiting with some friends from high school who sorta creep you out now but are fun to swap old stories with once a year. We'll get into maintenance next, but for now, know that as part of your motivation, you're free to start planning one big post-diet meal.

I had a small Midnight Truffle Blizzard from Dairy Queen (770 calories) the night before I flew to New Zealand. I could tell you it wasn't incredibly delicious, but I'd be lying. I could also tell you I didn't think about the calories in every single spoonful, but that'd be a lie, too. I enjoyed that Blizzard immensely, but I also knew deep down that it was a very rare fling with the forbidden. I was OK with that; you will be, too.

MAINTAINING

I've developed a new philosophy . . . I only dread one day at a time. —CHARLIE BROWN

HAVE YOU LOST THE WEIGHT YET? DON'T WORRY, YOU WILL soon. It'll be a wonderful accomplishment, something to take great pride in and to enjoy each and every day. But that doesn't mean you're done. The next phase is keeping it off, and you shouldn't underestimate the difficulty of that challenge.

It's daunting to know how few dieters are able to maintain their weight loss. A 2010 study in the *International Journal of Obesity,* using data from a survey of 14,000 people, found that only a slim majority of adults who had been overweight managed to keep any weight off. Among people who have lost 5 percent of their weight, only 36.5 percent managed to keep it off for at least a year. Only 4.4 percent of the people who responded were able to keep off 20 percent of their total weight. In total, about 20 percent of people who lost 10 percent of their weight or more could keep it off for a year. Depressing, right?

"It remains clear that the great majority of individuals who are overweight are not able to lose much weight and keep it off for the long term. This suggests that the majority of Americans will be unable to maintain a significant amount of weight loss without a significant change in either the efficacy or availability of weight loss and weight maintenance interventions," the authors wrote.

So the odds are against you. *Really against you.* Or they would be if you hadn't lost the weight using such a responsible, commonsense method—living your life in a way that's totally sustainable as you go forward, post-diet. And if you didn't have the information I'm about to share with you.

Here's the thing: You already know exactly what you need to do to maintain your weight indefinitely. Remember the Harris-Benedict equation we used to figure out what you'd need to eat to lose a pound per week? Obviously, it'll also tell you what you need to eat to keep your weight static. Your activity level may fluctuate a bit, but probably not enough to make a huge difference if you're counting your calories and limiting yourself to an exact amount every day. But, honestly, I don't count my calories every day—not unless I see myself put on a pound or two over a few weeks—and I'm not going to ask you to do that, either.

To figure out how to not get Re-Fat, we need to look at one big question: Why are other dieters so bad at keeping weight off?

It's a complicated question, one that a research project called the National Weight Control Registry has been examining for nearly twenty years now. This ongoing study, run out of Brown University's medical school, is open to anyone who has lost at least 30 pounds and maintained that loss for at least a year. Hopefully, if you had that much to lose when you started, you'll join me in registering very soon.

The registry does a great job of pointing out one undeniable fact: There are no easy solutions for keeping weight off. The main problem, scientists suppose, is that when your body has been overweight, it feels a pull to return to that weight. A weird tendency, I know, but one probably rooted back in those evolutionary cues to maintain extra energy stores in case of famine. I imagine your subconscious is thinking something like this: *Oh, no, my precious energy! Where did it go? I had a huge extra amount stored, but somehow it's all used up now! I want it back!*

Whatever the reason, if you've been overweight, studies show that your body tends to stimulate your appetite more than the body of someone who's always been thin, and it simultaneously signals the body to protect fat stores. In other words, your bastard subconscious and those stupid fucking glands are conspiring against you.

At the same time, for every pound of weight you lose, your BMR drops by about 8 calories per day. So as you get lighter, it gets harder to create the sort of deficit you need to lose weight. It's easy to eventually plateau and then creep back up. BOOM! Before you know it, you're Re-Fat and back to Chapter 1.

The *Los Angeles Times* summed up the situation perfectly by comparing it to debt: "Becoming overweight, in other words, is like being issued a credit card with an uncomfortably high balance that you'll probably end up paying off forever. Making sure the pounds stay off means pitting one's willpower against a swarm of biological processes involving the brain, hormones, metabolism, and fat storage."

So what's a Chubster to do? You can use lots of little tricks, which we'll outline below. You've done so much to get where you are, now that you're reaping the benefits, it's important not to backslide. But first, let's try the easy (*easier*, anyway) ways.

Keep Counting

This is the toughest but most obvious method. Hopefully you've grown to love—or at least appreciate—the ritual of counting calories throughout your diet. Probably, though, you still see it as something of a hassle, despite all the wonderful tricks and time-savers you learned a few chapters back.

Still, the NWCR shows that the people who successfully maintain their lower weight keep a close watch on what they're eating, many even counting their calories every day. That's a major commitment, I know, which is why I'm not usually one of those people. And it might not be necessary—it hasn't been for me most of the time. I did, however, make myself count for a month or two after I gained 3 pounds on a big California trip. Soon enough, the extra weight was gone. Then, just after Christmas, another 3 pounds snuck on, so I counted again until they were gone. I have noticed that the scale starts to creep up a pound or two when I stop counting—and that it doesn't when I do—so I've accepted that counting will always be part of my life. You're probably in the same boat.

My advice? Right now, set a ceiling at which counting ceases to be optional. My suggestion is 5 pounds—if you put that much on, start counting until it's off and continue for a few months afterward, too. Write it down if it'll help you be more honest with yourself.

Stay on the Scale

In order to maintain your weight, you need to keep a close watch on yourself. A majority of NWCR participants reported weighing themselves at least once a week, with a surprising 44 percent saying they weigh themselves at least *once a day.* That's a lot of scale time, I know, but it's also a way to keep weight at the front of your mind. Maybe you should hop on right before breakfast every day. Or maybe just do it every Sunday.

Either way, make sure you're stepping on the scale enough to always know where you are. If you do find yourself putting on a pound or two, it's a lot easier to buckle down and catch that than to try to lose 5 or 10 pounds you've unwittingly gained. Backsliding is rough: At a rate of 2 pounds a week, you're looking at more than a month to take off 10 pounds of Christmas cookies. All to get back to where you were just a short time ago. Not fun.

Exercise

Though researchers aren't sure how it all plays out under your skin, regular exercise is the most common trait shared by people who successfully maintain their weight loss. No, working out isn't the most effective way to actually peel pounds off—I belabored that point earlier—but once you've lost the weight, workouts really help keep it off. As researchers poring over the NWCR statistics have noted, successful maintainers tend to be "highly active," and a lot of success stories come from people who spend an hour or more each day in aerobic exercise. That sounds like a lot, but you won't necessarily have to do that. I work out for 45 minutes or so three or four times a week, which seems to do the trick.

Exercise helps dull your appetite, too. The exact mechanisms haven't quite been identified, but physical activity seems to cause your body to use certain hormones in a way that tampers down appetite, which may be another reason it's such a key element for people who manage to keep weight off.

Besides, if you do it right, exercise is fun. Walking, running, and the like are huge helpers when it comes to your mental health, so regular exercise is a great habit to establish. Maybe you should think of it this way: Would you rather run for a half-hour every few days or count every calorie you consume forever? Either option gives you a pretty solid chance of succeeding, so pick your poison!

Throw Out Your Old Clothes

I got rid of almost everything old and big in my closet, which has helped my maintenance plan tremendously. It's important to get rid of anything too large for you—especially the stopgap thrift store purchases you snagged mid-loss, which could provide a gentle ramp back to fatness. Rather than slowly slipping into larger and larger clothes—first into fat jeans, then off to the store to buy new jeans—I can tell if I'm at risk of putting on weight and adjust accordingly.

The fact that I wear the same T-shirt in different colors (the greatest shirts ever made, American Apparel 50/25/25 track shirts, if you're curious) three or four days a week helps a lot, too. After all, when all your shirts are the same, there's no risk of unconsciously drifting toward bigger and bigger items in your closet. If, like me, you really appreciate standardization in T-shirts, this is a great way to keep yourself in line.

Wear the Same Belt Every Day

Do you really need more than one belt? I don't—not unless it's a special occasion, anyway. So I wear my tooled leather belt with a solid brass Arizona Statehood 1912 buckle almost every day. And I still set it in the hole I punched when I dropped below 190. If I come out of that hole, I know I need to get my ass counting again.

Yeah, I know this one is more for the fellas than the ladies, since the fairer sex tends to feel a stronger commitment to a wider variety of clothing. Still, it's worked well for me, so I'm throwing it out there. Gentlemen: Find a belt and stick to it. You'll stay thin forever.

Refocus Your Culinary Quests

Maybe, like me, you want your food to be something of an adventure. Maybe you bring the spirit of a collector to the relatively simple act of feeding yourself, always keeping an eye out for the rare and wonderful. Maybe you've even planned your vacations around legendary restaurants.

That's me. In fact, I wrote the Wikipedia article on that shit. Quite literally, actually. If you dig around the Wikipedia article about the James Beard Foundation's America's Classics category (the world's snootiest foodies recognize a handful of legendary down-home mom-and-pop restaurants across the country every year), you'll see I originally compiled the information. It's the one and only time I've made a meaningful contribution to Wikipedia instead of, say, inserting "Franklin County Community College" into the list of common nicknames for An Ohio State University before the Michigan game.

Hey, I get it: Being snobby about food is fun. I've always gravitated to the best downscale foods around—I don't eat offal and I'm allergic to shellfish, so pricier delicacies are usually wasted on me—but I'm definitely down with culinary pretentiousness. It's fun to hunt down the best type of whatever food you're into. Used to be, I hearted pizza. I ate pizza at least a few times a week and was always looking for the next great place. I'd drive around town, checking out new places on other people's recommendations. When I went on a trip, I always asked around to find the best places wherever I was, maybe trying a handful over the course of a weekend on the road. I was pretty much the same way about beer—always looking for the best new or seasonal microbrew and sucking down whatever else I came across in the process.

I still like pizza and beer. Hell, I've priced tickets to Belgium to spend a few days hitting breweries, planning to sneak a case or two of Westvleteren, the world's best beer, made by monks and sold only at their abbey, back with me. But I've also found another, much healthier obsession: apples. There are about 7,500 cultivars of apple in the world—all descended from a wild species found in the 'Stans of Central Asia. In fact, since an apple has 57,000 genes, twice as many as a human, there are a lot of exotic types to search out. Even the worst grocery store in my hood will have at least a dozen types over the course of a year, which adds a little excitement to my shopping. When you get into all the organic and heirloom varieties too oddly shaped, tough-skinned, or bitter to make it to the masses but available on the farmer's market scene, there's a lot to try.

Have you had a SweeTango? That's the new cultivar from the University of Minnesota apple-breeding program that gave us Honeycrisp—and they're *amazing*. It's hard to find them even in season, and if you want to buy them online you're looking at $49.99 for a twelve-pack. Yet it'd almost be worth $4 per apple to me, they are that good. And they have only some 80 calories each.

See how I did that? You can do it too.

Eat Breakfast—and All the Other Meals, Too

As the same article in the *AJCN* points out, people who have successfully maintained their weight loss share one big eating habit in common: They eat breakfast. An astounding 78 percent of NWCR participants report eating breakfast every day of the week, while a meager 4 percent say they never eat breakfast. There's also at least some correlation with what they eat, with a typical breakfast being cereal and fruit.

A majority of NWCR participants also held themselves to the good old-fashioned three-meals-a-day thing, having a few snacks along with breakfast, lunch, and dinner every day. Staying on a routine is always a great way to continue any habit, and it seems to work very well with weight loss.

I'm pretty militant about my mealtimes—too much so, some have claimed. I eat breakfast (coffee and fibery cereal with a banana and maybe an apple if I'm superhungry) between 8 and 9 A.M. pretty much every day. Lunch is between noon and 1 P.M., and I start getting antsy if I haven't had dinner by 6 P.M. Not everyone needs to be so scripted about their mealtimes, but I find it helps me keep on track—and I'm far from alone.

Eat Low-Glycemic Foods

Back when silly low-carb diets were all the rage, a number of researchers tried to tackle the trend from various angles. One article in the *New England Journal of Medicine* found that people who ate a low-glycemic diet maintained their weight loss better than others.

Several diets are based on the glycemic index and Chubster isn't one of them, but since there is some evidence behind it as far as maintenance goes, I thought I'd mention it. You absolutely don't need another book, though. You can find everything you need to know about low-glycemic foods online, including a handy index that shows where broccoli and parsnips stack up against each other (broccoli is the clear winner). But for our purposes, just know that high-fiber foods like brown rice and rye bread and foods like cabbage, chickpeas, grapefruit, and yams tend to promote maintenance better than cornflakes, baguettes, and the like.

Stay Consistent

Think you can indulge a little extra at Sunday breakfast or on that Caribbean cruise you've been saving for? You might be able to, but a lot of people who are successful at maintaining their weight loss say they keep their diet consistent, regardless of whether it's a weekend or holiday.

Nearly 60 percent of NWCR participants said their eating habits were the same on weekends and weekdays, while nearly half (45 percent) said they did not cut themselves slack on holidays or vacation. Maybe you're the exception, but be careful here—you're playing with fire.

True story: I actually lost weight on a cruise. I was only three months into my diet at the time, true, but when my mother took my sister and me to Alaska, I managed to lose 2 pounds a week amid an inexhaustible supply of really tempting foods. My big secret? I avoided the buffets like the plague. Our ship had what I called "the Trough" upstairs and a nice little restaurant serving fish down below—I stayed belowdeck. I also went for frequent walks on the decks and read instead of ate. You can do that, too. Because, really, how much of a vacation is it if the best thing you can think to do is stuff your face?

I'll allow myself to run a calorie surplus on special occasions, like holidays where old family recipes are cooked or trips to places known for amazing food, but never for more than a few days at a time and nothing too extreme. Remember, the rules of mathematics mean that any surplus you run will eventually need to be countered by a deficit. There is no such thing as "cheating." When people understand the nature of that myth, they stop trying to game the system with an extra slice of pie because they know they'll have to make up for it later.

This, I think, is why more than half the people on NWCR never bother to indulge. When you know and accept at the very core of your being that you're not getting away with anything, it becomes much easier to just enjoy what you can in moderation instead of trying to sneak in a splurge. It's hard to make yourself accept that, I know. Especially in a culture that seems to be obsessed with selling people products that will magically allow them to break whatever rule they feel is holding them back. But that's how it is, folks.

Know That It Gets Easier

While the one-year figures for keeping weight off aren't necessarily encouraging for dieters, things do start to look better.

If you can make it to two years without regaining weight, you've got only about a 50 percent chance of relapse. So it gets easier. Every day you go without getting Re-Fat makes it a little easier, according to the studies. Someday—hopefully far, far into the future—you'll leave a skinny corpse.

The Principle of Limited Indulgence

So what does all this tell us? That it's important to maintain discipline but also that it's important to be flexible. Accountability—from a scale, from your clothing, from a record of what you've been eating—is the first key, since you can't successfully maintain something you're not watching. Then it's all about knowing when and where you can give yourself a little break and when to push yourself a little harder. Sure, it's a cliché— "All things are good in moderation"—but that doesn't make that Aristotelian concept any less true for dieters.

So have a piece of cake. Heck, have a Blizzard. Just don't do it all the time the way you did back when you were hamstringing your body with all that extra weight to begin with. Indulge as appropriate; limit as necessary.

The goal is something like personal sustainability. I hate to use that word, but it's the one that makes the most sense. Eat what you can eat without getting fat. It's easy to do that once you've unlocked the secrets of how your body uses what you put into it. That's what reading this book has been all about, right?

So that's pretty much it. Now you know what you need to know; you just need to make it happen. And you will—I have the utmost faith in you. Hell, after writing all this *for you*, I'd almost take it personally if you failed and got Re-Fat. It'd be like *we* were failing. Please, don't bring such shame upon me. Upon *us*. And don't bring all the things that come from obesity on yourself. There's no reason—no reason at all—not to lose the weight you need to lose to maintain a sustainable lifestyle.

It makes such a huge difference in every aspect of your life. There's so little to give up compared to all the wonderful things you ultimately get back in return. Such as not having your diabetes-ravaged leg chopped off, forcing a loved one to roll your ass around town as passersby look at you with pity.

You can still enjoy everything that plumped you up—you just need to do it in moderation and mix in more activities. Hey, as it turns out, even an evening Slurpee isn't off the table.

Remember the Slurpee that changed my life? The one I had on the way home from that awful Dave Matthews concert lo those many moons ago? The one that prompted the stern lecture from my girlfriend that, in turn, launched my weight-loss project?

Turns out, that Slurpee was the last one I had for nearly two years. Not that I stopped wanting them—I'm a sucker for pretty much any frozen confection and have always had a soft spot for the sweet, slushy treat favored by Bart Simpson. Since losing 100 pounds, I had allowed myself occasional indulgences of most types on limited occasions (see above), but never a Slurpee.

Then, one day, things came full circle.

South Mountain is the first Arizona mountain I ever stood atop. That's because it's the one peak you can drive up to. Like a lot of people in Phoenix, I would take out-of-town visitors up the narrow, saguaro-lined road up to the lookout so they could gaze down on our grid in all its suburban splendor. It's not a bad view.

One January evening, almost exactly a year after I'd achieved my goal weight for that New Zealand trip, I saw the reverse side of that drive.

Feeling a little burnt out on my favorite trails, I'd made a New Year's resolution to hike every route mapped out in Cosmic Ray's *Hiking Phoenix,* a crudely illustrated, self-published hiking bible written by a local hippie that's sold a staggering 100,000 copies.

I ended up on a brutal trail. Phoenix's South Mountain Park, at 25 square miles, is the largest city park in the country and bigger than Manhattan. Its Alta Trail is a steep route through some of the more isolated parts of the park. In fact, I only saw two people during a 4-hour hike, despite the fact that I was gazing down on the fifth-largest city in the country. Ol' Ray said the trail "really kicked [his] butt," but I figured I'd be able to do it in about half his 5-hour recommended time, the way I'd done with his other hikes. Nope. I set out on a 7-mile trail around 3 P.M. and wasn't close to finishing when the winter sun slipped behind the peaks to the west. I was out there nearly 2 more hours.

It was a hard hike. I was cold and surrounded by prickly things on a dark trail that had taken me at least a mile as the crow flies from the nearest soul. It was rough, and by the time I got to my car, I was ready for a cold drink from the closest convenience store.

So on my stop home I was lured into a 7-Eleven for a giant diet fountain soda. Instead, I found something I hadn't seen before: a Diet Slurpee.

Now, the Crystal Light Slurpee isn't calorie-free. There are actually 80 calories in a 16-ounce serving. But after hiking 7 long, steep miles, I was certainly willing to allow myself such a splurge.

Sitting in my car, savoring that slushy under a harsh neon glow while kids set off firecrackers behind the building, I thought back to the view I had on the trail. Coming down that trail in the dark, I looked across the valley to watch headlights wind their way up and down the road to the summit. It wouldn't be a bad road to suck down a 600-calorie Slurpee on, enjoying the view of the ocotillo and palo verde through the window of a car. That's one way to live, certainly. But the alternative is so much better. A little colder and a little lonelier on this particular night, but still so much more fulfilling than the things I'd experienced in my fat years. *That* was wasting; *this* is living.

Back at the beginning of this book, I made a reference to being "happily fat." And, truthfully, I enjoyed my run. But my life now is so, *so* much better. And not because I can swim at a public pool without being self-conscious or fit into a roller coaster or buy a T-shirt from any damned band I please. It's not the absence of all those little things I used to worry about; it's the presence of things I'd forgotten existed.

This is what I've come to realize: There are two ways up the mountain. You can drive up with 600 calories of sugary ice in your hand, or you can walk up and drink the artificially sweetened version. One route is wide, paved, and busy; the other, narrow, a little rocky, and far less crowded. One will give you little tastes of life as we were meant to live it from time to time; the other will immerse you in it fully. We all choose a path, consciously or not. Now, it's time for you to hop on the right one. It's time to make yourself a Chubster[2].

And really, how much will you miss gingerbread?

ACKNOWLEDGMENTS

CHUBSTER OWES ITS EXISTENCE TO A GREAT MANY PEOPLE, A few of whom I'd like to thank here.

Kirsten, my girlfriend, to whom this book is dedicated, for loving me enough to inspire me to lose 100 pounds and for being there through all the ups and downs along the way.

Brian, my BFF, who, in addition to being the best friend any guy could ask for, has edited approximately 1,000,000,000 of my words over the last decade and who helped mightily with this project, just as he's helped with everything I've done in my career.

Meagan, my editor at Houghton Mifflin Harcourt, who has great ideas and possesses a more perfect blend of enthusiasm and patience than any editor I've known.

Lindsay, my agent at Levine Greenberg, who saw the potential for this book in what now seems like a pretty messy proposal. I'm not sure why she wanted to waste her time representing an author who pitched a book with a chapter solely concerning how awesome Jared Fogle is, but I thank her for it.

My friends Dan Gibson and Shanna Hogan, who helped me figure out how to worm my way into the publishing industry. They have books for sale, too, and you should buy them.

My mother, sister, and father for constant support.

All the cool people I worked with at The Buchtelite, especially Art, Dan, Rob, Chad, Delano, the Lee sisters, Jon-O, and Katie. Everyone at *Akron Beacon Journal,* especially Char and Lynne. Everyone at the *Daily News-Record,* especially Cort, Katheryn, and Luanne. Everyone who worked at the *Old East Valley Tribune,* especially Jess and Noah.

And of course everyone I worked with at *Phoenix New Times,* especially Rick Barrs, Amy Silverman, Michael Lacy, Jay Bennett, and Jim King. If I go any further I'm sure to leave someone out, but thanks are deserved by almost everyone I worked with at *New Times* while writing this book.

(Not Benjamin.)

INDEX